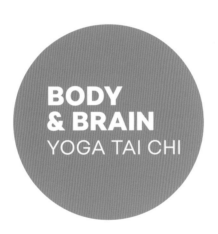

**BODY
& BRAIN**
YOGA TAI CHI

BEST LIFE MEDIA

459 N. Gilbert Road, Suite C-210
Gilbert, AZ 85234
www.BestLifeMedia.com
(480) 926-2480

First paperback edition: March 2020
Library of Congress Control Number:2019957841
ISBN-13: 978-1-947502-16-1

BODY&BRAIN YOGA EDUCATION

BODY & BRAIN
YOGA TAI CHI

A BEGINNER'S GUIDE
TO HOLISTIC WELLNESS

BEST
LIFE
MEDIA

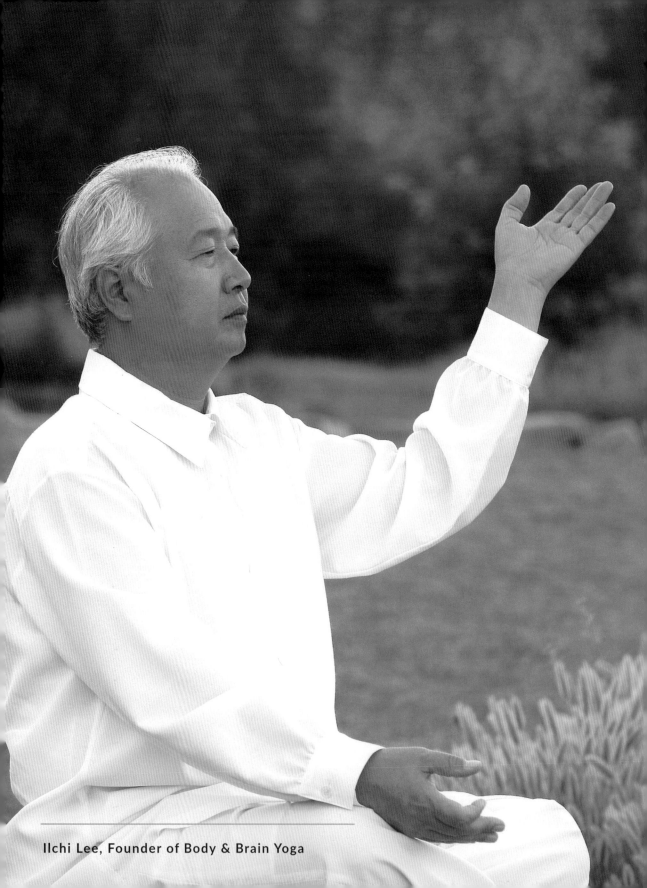

Ilchi Lee, Founder of Body & Brain Yoga

FOREWORD

"My body is not me, but mine."

This is a phrase that Body & Brain Yoga practitioners around the world speak with great enthusiasm. Its meaning has been central to the Body & Brain Yoga method since its beginnings in a small Korean park in the early 1980s. As the practice has developed into a global training method over the last 40 years, this phrase has continued to be an essential element in Body & Brain training.

The training techniques of Body & Brain Yoga are designed to develop mastership of the body and mind through the medium of energy, which is the means of communication between the body and mind. Through this process, you come to understand experientially the true meaning of the phrase, "My body is not me, but mine." Once this level of mastership has been achieved, you can apply this experience to the full spectrum of everyday life.

Since I first created Body & Brain Yoga, based on traditional Korean mind-body training methods, the basic philosophy and principles have not changed. But the training methods have been continuously improved. As humanity's understanding of the human body has increased, many people have tried to create an easier and more effective training system based on the experiences of Body & Brain Yoga instructors and their students. It has also been interwoven with modern research on the brain. This book is the result of those efforts.

One of the simplest and most effective concepts in Body & Brain Yoga is the idea of "breath." All living beings breathe. It is necessary for survival on this planet. However, most people take it for granted. Few people pay attention to their own breathing. But the quality of our breath has great implications for the health of our mind and body.

Whether we pay attention to our breath or choose to ignore it, we will continue to inhale and exhale. Through the experiential understanding of the breath achieved in Body & Brain Yoga training, the connection between mind-body communication and breath becomes more apparent.

Breath also dramatically demonstrates the interconnectedness of people. The air and energy that one person breathes in is the same air and energy that others have just breathed out. Being aware that everyone shares the same air cultivates the understanding that all living things are interconnected—not only through breath, but on many levels. Ultimately, this understanding helps develop more caring, open-hearted individuals and in turn creates a more harmonious world.

Imagine that a bell sits on the floor in front of you. No matter how great that bell is, if you don't ring it, there will be no sound. The same is true with Body & Brain Yoga. It is not a theory, but a practical way of life. Include Body & Brain Yoga as part of your daily practice and stick with it so that you can experience its full benefit. I sincerely hope that this book will help you take your first steps toward a healthier, happier, and more peaceful life.

Ilchi Lee
Founder of Body & Brain Yoga

TABLE OF CONTENTS

PART 1
THE
PRINCIPLES

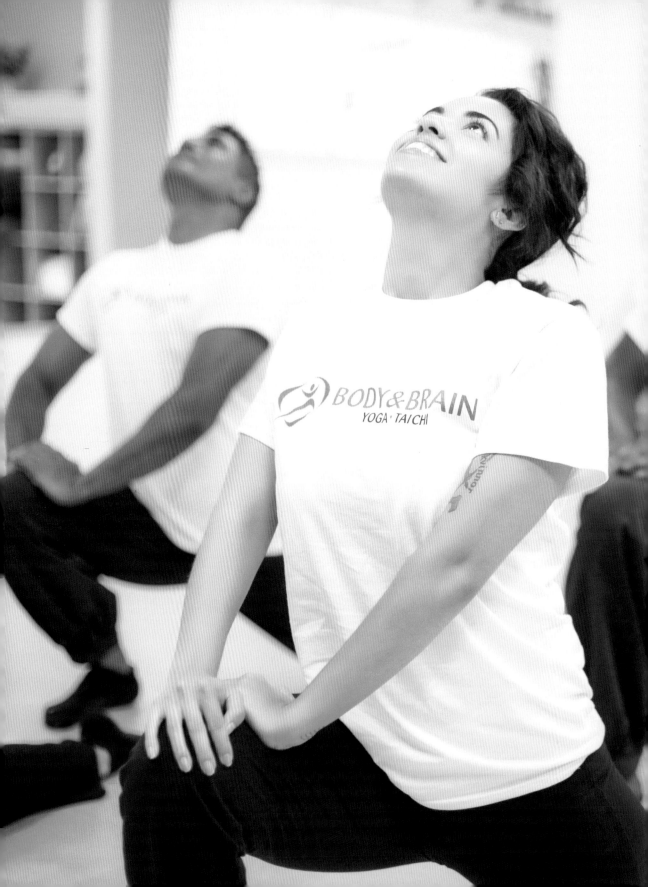

CHAPTER 1
WHAT IS BODY & BRAIN YOGA?

Body & Brain Yoga is an integrated mind-body training method that combines deep stretching exercises, meditative breathing techniques, vibration exercises, and energy awareness training. Body & Brain Yoga is a part of the Brain Education system of personal development created by Ilchi Lee. It helps practitioners achieve their greatest personal potential by strengthening the brain-body connection and developing self-mastery.

The traditional name for Body & Brain Yoga is *Dahnhak*, which literally means "the study of energy." In Korean, "*dahn*" refers to the primal, vital energy that is essential to all life forms, and "*hak*" refers to the study of a particular theory or philosophy. Thus, a Dahnhak practitioner is someone who studies the system of energy animating body and mind for the purpose of self-development.

What is energy? Energy connects body and mind, matter and consciousness, from the personal level all the way to the cosmic level. The nature and actions of energy have been studied and used for thousands of years in Eastern cultures for personal development and holistic wellness. During Body & Brain Yoga training, practitioners learn how to use these principles to heal and develop strength of body, mind, and spirit for optimal holistic health. The most commonly recognized benefits include increased vitality, focus, and capacity to manage stress, as well as emotional balance and a positive attitude. Essentially, Body & Brain Yoga practitioners can regain mastership over their bodies and brains by incorporating an awareness of energy into their exercises.

The benefits of Body & Brain Yoga extend beyond personal health and wellness, as positive changes in one's physical, mental, and emotional condition also affect other aspects of life. People often report that as they practice Body & Brain Yoga, their family life improves, they gain confidence in their career, and they are even able to release the burdensome emotional baggage of old relationships.

As practitioners move toward the goal of creating a healthier personal life, they often develop the power and willingness to foster more harmonious relationships with family, friends, communities, and the natural world. This, in turn, helps them develop their personal capabilities in a way that contributes to a healthier, happier, and more peaceful world.

Where Did It All Begin?

The roots of Body & Brain Yoga extend back several thousand years to a Korean philosophy and mind-body practice known as *Sundo*. Sundo was designed to educate the Korean population to develop character as well as strength and intelligence. This practice, also known as "the path of enlightenment," was followed daily to help maintain health and develop one's potential as an ideal human being. Up until 2,000 years ago, Sundo was widely practiced and transmitted from one generation to the next, contributing to the health and unity of the Korean people for many hundreds of years. However, in the face of multiple invasions by foreign countries and the suppression of the original Korean culture, the Sundo tradition was forgotten. It became an esoteric practice known to only a few.

During his personal journey toward self-realization, Ilchi Lee rediscovered the essence of the Sundo tradition and modernized it. Lee first taught it in 1980 to a stroke patient he met in a small park in Anyang, South Korea. Others soon heard about this informal class and sought to join and learn Ilchi Lee's techniques and philosophies. As a result, the first official training center was opened in 1985. Its popularity grew steadily, and in 1996, the practice was introduced in the United States. It has now expanded throughout the world, with more than 600 centers offering Body & Brain Yoga to more than 200,000 active practitioners. In addition, the practice is taught at thousands of public parks, schools, worksites, assisted living centers, and college campuses in South Korea, the United States, Canada, Japan, the United Kingdom, and other countries.

What Are the Benefits?

Body & Brain Yoga was created for people who want to utilize the wisdom of ancient mind-body practices while living active modern lives. One of the advantages of Body & Brain Yoga techniques is that they are easy and simple enough for anyone to learn, yet beneficial to even the most advanced practitioner. Anyone— regardless of age, gender, or experience level—can benefit from Body & Brain Yoga. Regular practice offers the following benefits:

FOR YOUR BODY

Breathing techniques, deep stretching movements, and body awareness training combine to work every muscle, joint, and organ in the body to help you:

- Improve energy and blood circulation.
- Increase flexibility and balance.
- Improve bone density and muscle tone.
- Help maintain a balanced metabolism.
- Promote cardiovascular health.
- Help manage pain in the body.

FOR YOUR MIND

Body & Brain Yoga helps you create an optimal energy balance and a physiological foundation for your brain's best performance. Body & Brain Yoga's integrated approach to developing the whole brain can help you:

- Relax and handle stressful situations more easily.
- Quiet the mind and improve concentration.
- Experience more positive thoughts and self-acceptance.
- Feel centered and balanced.
- Develop a sense of ownership of your health, happiness, and peace.

FOR YOUR SPIRIT

In addition to supporting physical and mental well-being, Body & Brain Yoga is uniquely designed to enhance the spiritual aspect of human existence. Body & Brain Yoga practice promotes a sense of peace and centeredness that can help you:

- Become more aware of your body, your feelings, and the world around you.
- Feel whole and connected with humanity and nature.
- Identify your life purpose and rekindle your passion for life.

What Makes Body & Brain Yoga Different?

Body & Brain Yoga is distinguished by three unique characteristics:

ENHANCING THE BODY-BRAIN CONNECTION

Body & Brain Yoga is based on the idea that the brain is the command center for the whole human body and its energy system. Through various Body & Brain Yoga programs, practitioners can learn principles and exercises designed to activate the brain's power to create a healthier, happier life for themselves and others. We all know that the human brain has the power to create conflict and intolerance in the world. Body & Brain Yoga maintains that the brain also has the power to create a healthier and more peaceful society.

THE MASTERY AND USE OF ENERGY

Because energy is the medium that connects body and mind, it is a defining characteristic of every Body & Brain Yoga exercise. Practitioners can develop a deeper understanding of their bodies and minds and strengthen communication between the two by directly experiencing this energy.

Practitioners first learn how to feel and accumulate energy in the major energy centers of the body. As the sense of energy gradually develops, formerly blocked energy channels open up, promoting energy circulation throughout the body. After developing the ability to control and command energy, people often experience natural healing as well as better management of their habits and emotions.

It is possible to follow Body & Brain Yoga training without feeling energy. However, with a sense of energy, practitioners can experience the true character of Body & Brain Yoga as a joyful and multidimensional experience.

SELF-MANAGED, HOLISTIC HEALTH

In addition to being good for the body, Body & Brain Yoga includes principles and techniques that support a sense of ownership of one's emotional health. As empowered owners of their own minds, Body & Brain Yoga practitioners naturally seek to manage their physical and emotional habits. This extends to managing social interactions and developing healthy communication skills as well as correcting unhealthy habits, such as smoking and overeating. The key principles of Body & Brain Yoga and its systematic training methods make all of this possible, as will be explained in greater detail later in this book.

"Feel the bright energy inside you and develop it through practice. Design your life using that bright energy."

—*Ilchi Lee*

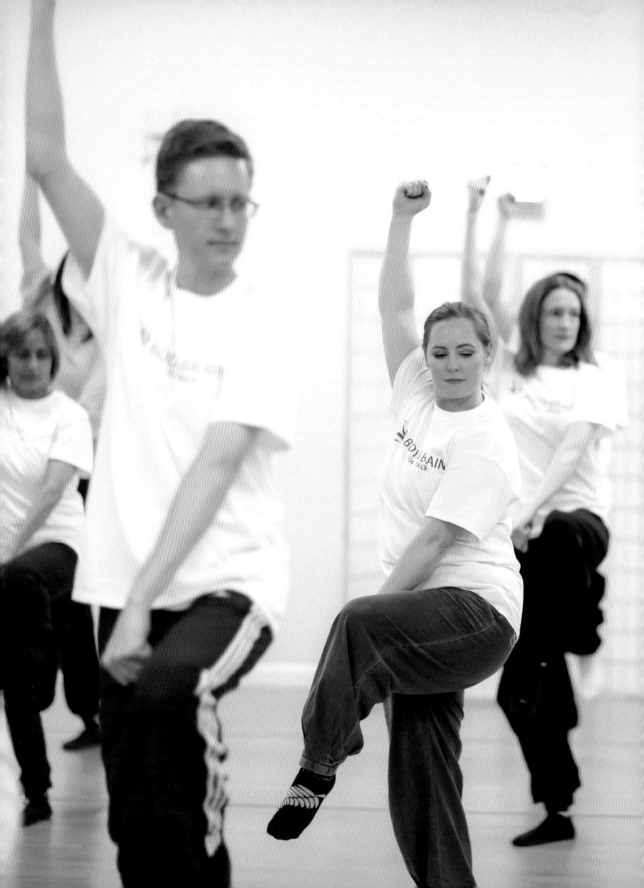

CHAPTER 2

THE PHILOSOPHY AND PRINCIPLES OF BODY & BRAIN YOGA

The Philosophy

The core philosophy of Body & Brain Yoga is based on Brain Education, Ilchi Lee's practical system of personal development, which combines the ancient Korean tradition of mind-body training known as Sundo with modern neuroscientific understanding.

SUNDO PHILOSOPHY

Among the key concepts passed down from Sundo and incorporated into Brain Education and Body & Brain Yoga are oneness with nature, a mastery of energy, living as one's true self, and the spirit of *Hongik*, a Korean word that translates to "widely benefiting."

Sundo training methods aim to create a state of harmony in which humans and nature are one. Sundo suggests that the human body and brain have the power to maintain their own health when allowed to follow their natural rhythms. Sundo practice eliminates or transforms disruptions to these rhythms, such as stress and tension, inadequate circulation, toxin buildup, harmful thoughts, and emotional trauma. By achieving a state of internal harmony and balance, we can live in harmony with our true self, other people, and nature.

The Five Steps of Brain Education

Once you understand how your BOS works, you can begin using it to manage your brain. Brain Education lays out a five-step process for this. By following this process, you will become more aware of your body and brain and learn to use them effectively to achieve your goals. You will be able to better coordinate your brain functions to enhance your health, happiness, and peace, and you will enjoy challenging your brain with new situations and perspectives. Brain Education is designed to create a Power Brain—a brain that is productive, creative, and peaceful.

To achieve the personal growth that you desire, it's important to continuously practice all five steps of Brain Education. Over time, you'll notice your ability and awareness expanding. Each Body & Brain Yoga class and workshop will help you experience the following five steps more fully.

STEP 1: BRAIN SENSITIZING

Become aware of your body's senses and energy. Strengthen the connection between your body and your brain, and experience what an optimal energy balance feels like. Increase your ability to be mindful and present in each moment.

STEP 2: BRAIN VERSATILIZING

Release stress and stretch your body and brain to make them more flexible. Your brain's neuroplasticity lets you respond to change and challenges with a resilient and adaptable mindset. Become someone who welcomes and uses change with a positive and confident attitude.

STEP 3: BRAIN REFRESHING

Refresh your brain by freeing it from unhelpful thoughts and emotions and empowering it with positive information. Change your perspective and see new possibilities and potential.

STEP 4: BRAIN INTEGRATING

Increase your brain power by engaging your whole brain. Coordinate your thoughts, words, and actions to align with your purpose so that your whole brain is working in harmony for health, happiness, and peace. Affirm what your true self wants, and then take action to achieve it.

STEP 5: BRAIN MASTERING

Create the life you want by systematically applying the first four steps of Brain Education in your daily life. Live a Hongik life and express your true self with passion and purpose.

THE FIVE STEPS OF
BRAIN EDUCATION

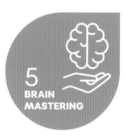

5 BRAIN MASTERING

- Empowers authorship of life purpose.
- Enables greater executive control of the brain.
- Expedites decision-making.

4 BRAIN INTEGRATING

- Unites different brain areas.
- Enhances communication between brain hemispheres.
- Releases latent abilities.

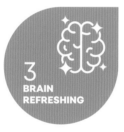

3 BRAIN REFRESHING

- Clears emotional residue.
- Encourages positive life view.
- Develops emotional intelligence.

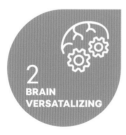

2 BRAIN VERSATALIZING

- Creates flexibility in brain circuitry.
- Frees brain from rigid habits.
- Opens mind to new information.

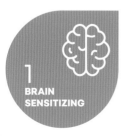

1 BRAIN SENSITIZING

- Awakens the five senses.
- Improves physiological functioning.
- Encourages brain awareness.

The Three Studies of Body & Brain Yoga

To understand and fully utilize Body & Brain Yoga, study the principles behind this practice and apply them in your everyday life.

Body & Brain Yoga is comprised of three studies: the study of principle, the study of practice, and the study of living. These should be done simultaneously and continuously, as each study supports and is supported by the others. By being mindful of these, you can live your life as an expression of the true Hongik spirit.

Here's how the three studies can help you benefit more fully from your Body & Brain Yoga practice.

THE STUDY OF PRINCIPLE

By learning the principles of Brain Education and the human energy system, you will understand how and why Body & Brain Yoga exercises work. This will help you stay motivated and practice correctly and efficiently for maximum benefit.

THE STUDY OF PRACTICE

Deepen your understanding of Brain Education principles by experiencing their effects on your body and mind through the practice of Body & Brain Yoga.

THE STUDY OF LIVING

Embody Brain Education and Body & Brain Yoga by using their principles and practices to improve your everyday life.

"Your brain is designed to help you find happiness. All you have to do is let it."

—*Ilchi Lee*

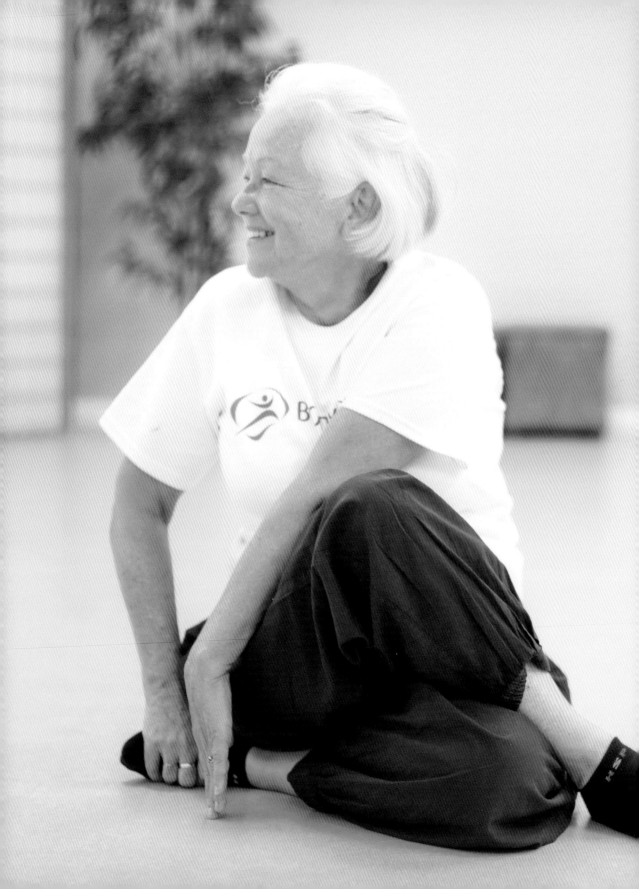

CHAPTER 3
THE VISION OF BODY & BRAIN YOGA

Individual Completion and Collective Completion

Body & Brain Yoga is a powerful practice for developing health, happiness, and peace. No matter where you're starting from, you can increase your flexibility and strength, develop greater self-awareness and concentration, and enjoy more confidence and creation power.

Ultimately, Body & Brain Yoga has the mission of helping people live complete lives—physically, emotionally, and spiritually. Reaching this state is known as individual completion. Helping humanity as a whole to reach this state is collective completion.

Individual completion means awakening to one's true self and achieving unity with the natural flow of the universe. Finding and growing the true self is accomplished through the study of principle, practice, and living. Through these three studies, the Hongik spirit of the true self emerges.

Naturally, as our capability to create health, happiness, and peace in our own lives grows, we look to share these things with those around us. Our study of living first expands from helping ourselves to helping our families, then to helping our communities and countries, and finally to helping all life on earth. As our practice deepens, our true self power expands, and our ability to care for everything expands along with it. This is how individual completion, or enlightenment, leads to a life of contribution and collective completion.

Empowering people to live a Hongik life is one of the fundamental goals of Body & Brain Yoga. Through group classes, workshops, retreats,

27

and personal practice, practitioners gain the experience necessary to share princi-ples and exercises with others. Many feel empowered to teach in their communi-ties at parks, schools, community centers, health centers, prisons, shelters, work-places, and more.

Such outreach activities began with founder Ilchi Lee. His first efforts to help people realize their own health and happiness started in a small local park in South Korea in 1980. Since then, thousands of people in several countries have continued this tradition, which has been formalized in the United States into the nonprofit Body & Brain Foundation.

Body & Brain Yoga centers and practitioners also support other nonprofits that share Brain Education for the greater good. These various organizations, such as the IBREA Foundation, not only have programs in countries where centers exist, but in developing countries as well.

Sharing what you learn through Body & Brain Yoga is a way to deepen your understanding of the practice, strengthen your confidence and action power, and brighten your Hongik spirit—which is the essence of a life of completion.

The Earth Citizen Movement

A person whose empathy and compassion has grown to encompass the whole planet has been named an "Earth Citizen" by Body & Brain Yoga founder Ilchi Lee. Earth Citizens are stewards of the Earth who want to manage the planet's resources for the benefit of all life. They put their identity as citizens of the entire globe before their national, cultural, or religious identities.

Earth Citizens endeavor to bring happiness and peace to the world and protect the balance of the Earth's natural environment. They grow their true selves and live according to the values of those true selves to create a new "Earth Citizen culture" based on respect for the Earth and all humanity. By taking on an Earth Citizen identity and values—Hongik values—we can help create health, happiness, and peace for one another and for the entire planet.

Ilchi Lee began the Earth Citizen Movement to raise awareness of the need for people to take on an Earth Citizen identity in order to have peace and prosperity on Earth. For many practitioners, an Earth Citizen identity arises naturally through the practice of Body & Brain Yoga. That's why many practitioners participate in Earth Citizen Movement activities and projects—such as teaching mind-body exercises in their communities, learning organic farming and an eco-friendly lifestyle, and hosting community festivals and walks for spreading Earth Citizen awareness. They also support the Earth Citizens Organization (ECO), a nonprofit that uses Brain Education to train Earth Citizen community leaders.

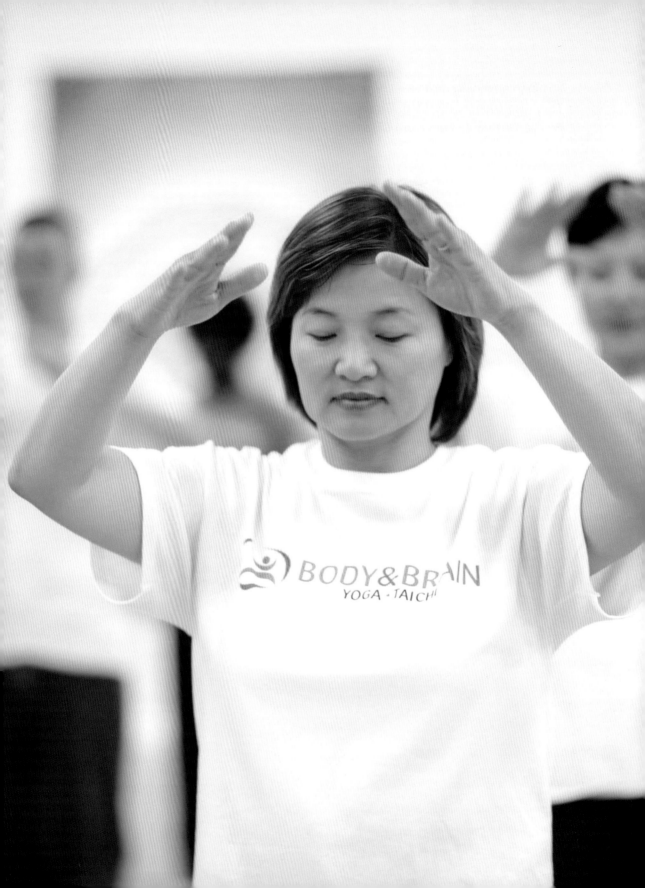

CHAPTER 4
THE ENERGY SYSTEM OF THE BODY

Ki, the Energy of Life

Ki—also spelled *chi* or *qi*—is a fundamental concept in Asian philosophy, arts, medicine, and mind-body traditions. Ki is the vital energy that is the true essence of every creation in the cosmos. Ideally, ki flows freely according to the rhythm of life, coming together and then dispersing. When ki amasses and condenses, it creates the forms of life we can see. Everything around us, as well as our very lives, are temporary manifestations of ki.

Most people first experience ki as the bioenergy that is the basic life force in the body. Beyond that, ki is also the bridge connecting body and mind. Human beings have an innate ability to sense ki, but an overdependence on rational thought and language often eclipses this sense. However, we can awaken this "sixth sense." In Body & Brain Yoga, we do this through the power of concentration and by using exercise and meditation to open blockages in the body's energy pathways. As these pathways open, we are able to make use of the information that is transmitted on energy pathways. Being able to feel ki gives us the ability to use and manage energy to recover and maintain our natural health and balance. Through an awareness of ki, we can more fully manifest the potential of our bodies and brains.

Jinki, the Energy of the Mind

There are three types of ki energy in the human body. *Wonki*, which means "primal energy," is the energy that you've inherited, or were born with. *Jungki*—"vital energy"—is the energy that you get by eating and breathing. *Jinki*, or "authentic energy," is generated through deep, concentrated breathing. Wonki and jungki are generated without conscious participation, while jinki requires focus. The energy developed in Body & Brain Yoga is jinki.

Since jinki is generated by the mind through concentration, its quality varies according to the state of the mind at any given time. A positive mental and emotional state produces a more positive energy. This, in turn, has a calming and relaxing effect on the body. A negative mental and emotional state has the opposite effect. When the flow of jinki is blocked or impeded by negative thoughts and emotions, the body becomes tense, resulting in stagnant energy.

We often use the concepts of *chunjikiun* and *chunjimaeum* in Body & Brain Yoga practice. Chunjikiun is another name for cosmic energy, or heaven and earth energy. In Korean, this means the highest level of ki that circulates throughout the universe. We experience chunjikiun when we have chunjimaeum—cosmic mind or "enlightened consciousness."

Energy Channels

Ki is transported throughout the body in a series of channels known as meridians. Meridians are like a system of canals carrying sustenance to body, mind, and spirit. Just as goods can be transported along waterways or roads, energy can be supplied to the organs and different parts of the body through the meridians. If energy flows well through the meridians, it is distributed evenly throughout the body, helping both body and brain maintain optimal condition.

Your body consists of 12 major meridians, each associated with one of the principal internal organs and named accordingly. These 12 meridians are paired, or bilateral, and positioned symmetrically on either side of the body. Body & Brain Yoga practice helps energy flow more freely throughout them.

Besides the 12 major meridians, your body has eight "extra" meridians. In Body & Brain Yoga practice, two of these are considered important. One is the Governing Vessel meridian (*Dokmaek* in Korean), which runs along the midline of the back; the other is the Conception Vessel meridian (*Immaek*), which runs along the front midline of the body. These two meridians meet at the junction of the lips.

RELATIONSHIP BETWEEN BODY, MIND & KI

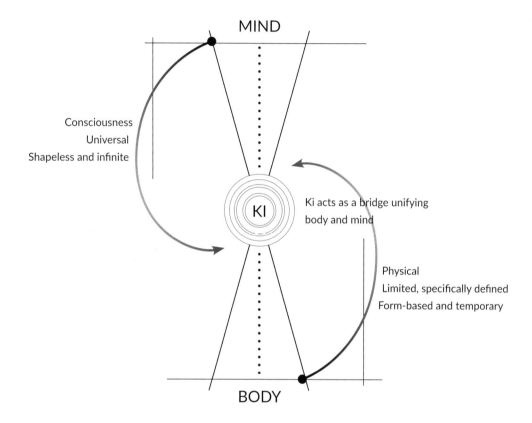

MIND

Consciousness
Universal
Shapeless and infinite

KI

Ki acts as a bridge unifying
body and mind

Physical
Limited, specifically defined
Form-based and temporary

BODY

A HAND OF A KI PRACTITIONER

The Kirilian energy photo on the left shows
a hand in a normal state. The picture on the
right shows the same hand emitting ki.

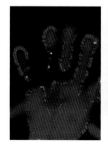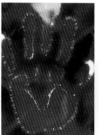

MERIDIANS: ENERGY CHANNELS

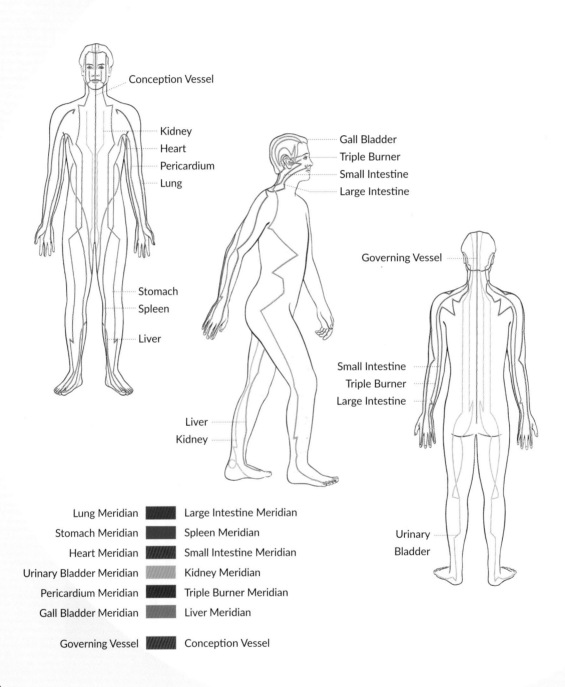

Conception Vessel

Kidney
Heart
Pericardium
Lung

Gall Bladder
Triple Burner
Small Intestine
Large Intestine

Governing Vessel

Stomach
Spleen

Liver

Small Intestine
Triple Burner
Large Intestine

Liver
Kidney

Urinary
Bladder

Lung Meridian   Large Intestine Meridian
Stomach Meridian   Spleen Meridian
Heart Meridian   Small Intestine Meridian
Urinary Bladder Meridian   Kidney Meridian
Pericardium Meridian   Triple Burner Meridian
Gall Bladder Meridian Liver Meridian

Governing Vessel   Conception Vessel

Energy Points

Along the meridians are points through which energy enters and exits the body, just as passengers enter and exit at stations along a train line. These points also serve as energy storage and distribution centers. The energy at a particular point tends to go to the organs and body parts associated with that point. These energy points are used in acupressure and acupuncture and are often called acupressure points or acupuncture points.

Besides gathering and transmitting energy, energy points send signals to the brain. Tenderness or pain at an acupressure point indicates an energy blockage that corresponds with an imbalance in the body. Stimulating that point informs the brain of the imbalance so that it can begin to repair it.

There are 365 primary energy points in the human body. The following are the most important in Body & Brain Yoga training.

BAEKHWE

Located at the top of the head, at the intersection of an imaginary line connecting the ears and another line connecting the spine and nose. *Baekhwe* literally means "100 energy points meeting." Sometimes called "Great Cosmic Gate," this is a major energy point through which energy is taken into the body during Body & Brain Yoga practice.

JUNJUNG

Located about one-and-a-half to two inches in front of the Baekhwe, *Junjung* is named "Small Cosmic Gate."

INDANG

Frequently called "the third eye," located between the eyebrows. When this point is activated, one might exhibit heightened intuition and extrasensory perception.

INJOONG

Located in the center of the valley between the nose and the lips. *Injoong* means "middle of a person."

OKCHIM

Two separate energy points, an inch to either side of the slightly protruding point at the back of the head.

NOEHO

Found at the very back of the head, in the center of where the skull protrudes most.

TAEYANG

Located on the temples, between the eyes and the tops of the ears. These are important activation points related to the brain.

AHMUN

Found between the first and second vertebrae, where the neck and head meet.

DAECHU

Located just below the seventh cervical vertebrae at the base of the back of the neck. Also called "Great Hammer" in English, it's important for colds and the flu.

DAHNJOONG

Located in the center of the slight indentation on the sternum.

JOONGWAN

Located halfway between the solar plexus and the navel.

SHINGWOL

Located exactly at the navel. *Shingwol* means "palace of God."

MYUNGMUN

Located on the back directly opposite the navel, between the second and third lumbar vertebrae. *Myungmun* means "the gate of life."

KIHAE

Located two inches below the navel, *Kihae* means "the sea of ki energy."

HWE-EUM

Located at the perineum (the base of the pelvis).

JANGSHIM

Located on each hand at the center of the palm. To find the *Jangshim* point, make a fist. The point is where the middle finger touches the palm.

YONGCHUN

Located on each foot at the center of the sole, one-third of the way down from the top of the toes.

IMPORTANT ENERGY POINTS

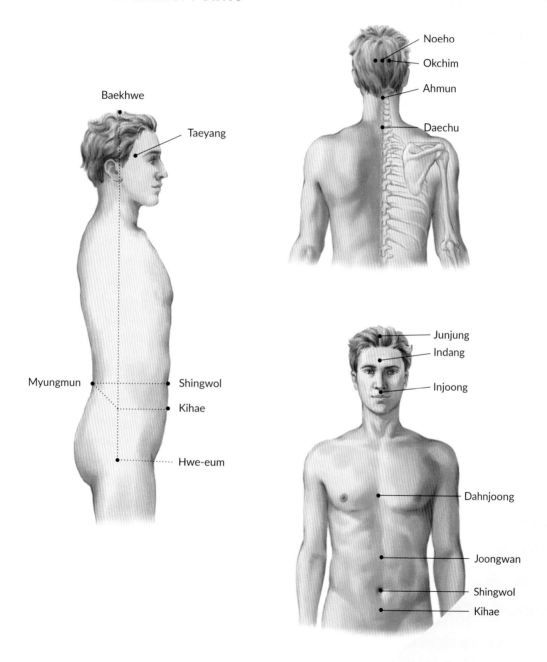

Baekhwe

Taeyang

Noeho

Okchim

Ahmun

Daechu

Myungmun

Shingwol

Kihae

Hwe-eum

Junjung

Indang

Injoong

Dahnjoong

Joongwan

Shingwol

Kihae

Energy Centers

The centers where large concentrations of energy are gathered and stored are another important component of the body's energy system. Although they don't exist on a physical level, energy centers can be thought of as the organs of the system. In Korean, these energy centers are called *dahnjons*, which translates as "fields of energy." Essentially, dahnjon has a similar meaning to the word chakra, which means "wheel" or "circle" in Sanskrit. Through Body & Brain Yoga, which enhances your ability to sense energy, you can feel energy gathering in a dahnjon.

If a dahnjon is blocked or weakened and the energy flow is disrupted, this may be manifested as a physical problem. Body & Brain Yoga exercises and breathwork can help facilitate the flow and power of energy through the dahnjons, resulting in more balanced energy and better overall health.

Body & Brain Yoga focuses on the development of three internal dahnjons and four external dahnjons. The internal dahnjons are in the abdomen, chest, and head. They correspond to three of the seven chakras thought to exist in the body. These chakras begin at the base of the trunk of the body and run along the spine. The last one, the seventh chakra, is found at the crown of the head. They have corresponding areas near the front of the body that can be used to sense and stimulate each chakra. Like the three dahnjons, chakras affect all aspects of physical, mental, and emotional wellness.

Relating to the second chakra, the lower dahnjon is in the lower abdomen, about two inches below the navel and two inches inside, behind the Kihae energy point. The middle dahnjon is in the center of the chest around the fourth chakra, behind the Dahnjoong point, while the upper dahnjon is in the center of the head. It corresponds to the sixth chakra. The four external dahnjons are located on each palm (*Jangshim*) and on the bottom of each foot (*Yongchun*).

The three internal dahnjons are defined by the roles they play. **The lower dahnjon** acts as a fuel tank, storing physical energy for circulation throughout the body. It also serves as a kind of furnace that converts the fuel into vitality and action power. When your lower dahnjon is strong, your body's vital energy is enhanced and balanced, and its natural healing power is optimized. You exhibit physical strength, patience, and drive, along with a firm sense of self-confidence. Red is the color associated with the lower dahnjon.

The middle dahnjon is associated with mastery of emotional energy. Strengthening the middle dahnjon helps cultivate a peaceful and loving feeling. Conversely, negative emotions and stress can suppress the energy flow of the middle dahnjon,

KEY ENERGY CENTERS (DAHNJONS)

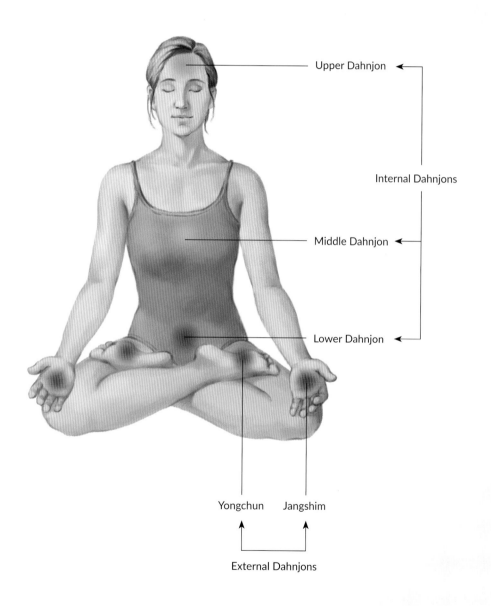

Upper Dahnjon

Internal Dahnjons

Middle Dahnjon

Lower Dahnjon

Yongchun   Jangshim

External Dahnjons

which can put stress on the nervous system and potentially contribute to many illnesses. The color of the middle dahnjon is golden yellow or green.

The upper dahnjon is related to spiritual and intellectual characteristics. When the upper dahnjon is strong, so is your clarity, intuition, creativity, and spiritual perception. You have a broader perspective and feel a connection with the divine energy of the cosmos. Blue-violet is the color associated with the upper dahnjon.

Our Three Bodies

While you are familiar with your physical body, you may not have heard of your other "bodies." In Body & Brain Yoga, it is said that we have three bodies representing three important aspects of our being: a physical body, an energy body, and a spiritual body. Each of these bodies is managed by one of the dahnjons. The lower dahnjon manages the physical body; when it is strong and full, the physical body is healthy. The middle dahnjon manages the energy body; when it is open and mature, emotions are stable and positive. The upper dahnjon manages the spiritual body, consisting of all of the information in the conscious and subconscious minds; when it is clear and bright, our intuition, perception, creativity, and decision-making abilities are fully manifested.

Rather than functioning independently, these three bodies are interconnected, with energy acting as the communication medium between them. Learning how to manage the three bodies and the energy system as a whole is an essential part of Body & Brain Yoga practice.

THE SEVEN CHAKRAS

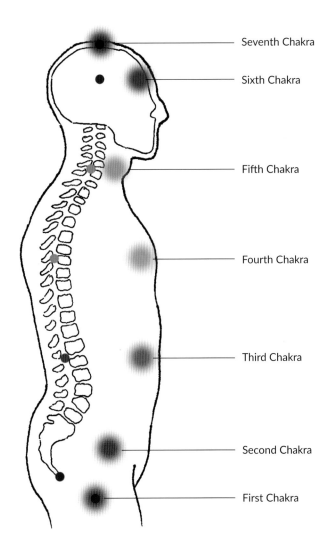

Seventh Chakra

Sixth Chakra

Fifth Chakra

Fourth Chakra

Third Chakra

Second Chakra

First Chakra

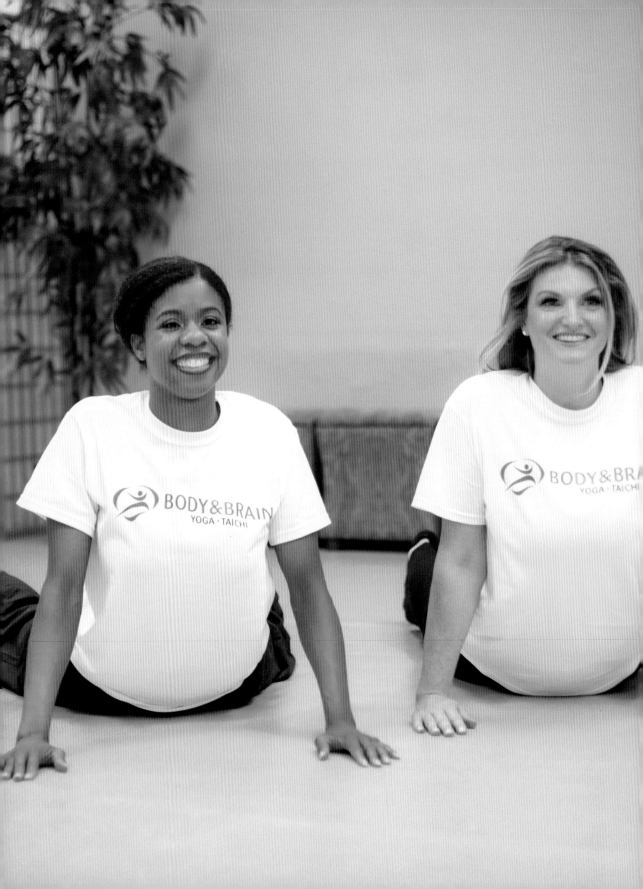

CHAPTER 5

THE ENERGY PRINCIPLES OF BODY & BRAIN YOGA

Now that you've seen the energy system of the human body, it's important to understand the basic natural principles by which that energy flows and operates. These principles form the basis for the stretching, breathing, and meditation techniques you'll experience in each Body & Brain Yoga class. Knowing these principles will help you make the most out of the practice and apply it to your everyday life.

The Three Energy Principles

WATER UP, FIRE DOWN

Within the energy system of our bodies, we have cool water energy and hot fire energy. When the energy system is in balance, cool water energy travels up toward the head while hot fire energy flows down to the lower abdomen. This natural circulation of energy is called Water Up, Fire Down, or *Suseung Hwagang* in Korean. This is the most important energy principle for optimal human health.

Water Up, Fire Down is similar to phenomena found in natural systems, such as the earth's water cycle. When fire energy from the sun reaches the earth, it heats up the rivers, lakes, and oceans, causing water energy to rise and form clouds. Plants exhibit this cycle, too, receiving fire energy from the sun while drawing water energy up through their roots. Within this cycle of energy, they grow and bear fruit. In winter, when days are shorter, the light from the sun is weaker, and the ground is too frozen for plants to bring up water, leaves fall to the ground and no fruit is produced. Growth is suspended until the natural cycle of energy resumes once more in the spring. Through Water Up, Fire Down energy circulation, life maintains balance and continuity.

In the human body, the kidneys and heart facilitate this natural circulation of energy with the help of the lower dahnjon. The heart generates fire energy, which descends along the front of the body to the lower dahnjon, where it is stored. Some of this accumulated warm energy travels to the kidneys, where it stimulates water energy to rise up along the spine to the head and cool the brain, pushing hot energy down to the heart and all the way down to the lower dahnjon.

When water energy reaches the brain, it creates a cool and refreshed feeling. And when fire energy comes down from the head and the heart, the abdomen and the organs inside it become warm and flexible. These positive effects are expressed in such common sayings as "Keep a cool head" and "I have a fire in my belly." When Water Up, Fire Down is in effect, your senses are opened and you can perceive with greater clarity of mind. You feel positive and relaxed, and you experience a greater sense of vitality and well-being. Your creativity and imagination are also enhanced.

If the Water Up, Fire Down energy flow is reversed and fire energy moves upward while water energy moves downward, then the abdomen may become clammy, cold, and tense. You may feel "weak at heart" or fatigued. In this state, many people experience digestive problems, including chronic constipation and tenderness in the abdomen. Some also encounter circulatory problems, reproductive or menstrual issues, or hormone imbalances. The fire energy rising to your head may make you feel "hot-headed" or stuck in a brain fog, with an overactive mind, trouble focusing, headaches, a stiff neck and shoulders, or a feeling of heaviness in your head.

There are two common circumstances in which Water Up, Fire Down is reversed or blocked. The first occurs when the lower dahnjon, which pulls in and stores energy, is weak or inefficient. In this case, fire energy collects in the head instead of going to the lower dahnjon, instigating a flurry of thoughts and emotions. Stress, manifested as too much energy stuck in the chest, can also interrupt Water Up, Fire Down. In this case, the fire energy in the heart is blocked by the buildup of energy in the chest. Instead of flowing downward, it backs up into the head. This can cause nervousness and anxiety.

WATER UP, FIRE DOWN

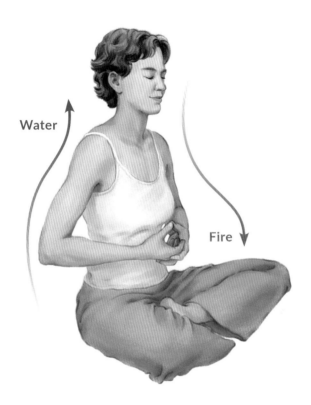

Water

Fire

Water Up, Fire Down (Healthy State)	Fire Up, Water Down (Unhealthy State)
Circulation, dynamic, lively	Disconnected, static, lifeless
Sweet saliva in the mouth	Dry mouth, bitter taste
Warm hands and feet	Cold hands and feet
Cool and refreshed head	Heat and pain in the head
Warm abdomen filled with energy	Abdomen lacks warmth and energy
Regular bowel movements	Constipation, digestive problems
Refreshed and energized	Tired and uncomfortable

Body & Brain Yoga exercises are designed to help relieve stress and tension in the chest and abdomen and strengthen the lower dahnjon so that Water Up, Fire Down circulation can be maintained for optimal health.

Energy, Meet Physiology

Water Up, Fire Down forms the basis for many Body & Brain Yoga exercises. But how does modern science reconcile this principle?

Consider many of the phenomena that are commonly associated with the development of Water Up, Fire Down: the abdomen warming, heart rate lowering, eyes tearing, and mouth watering. All of these sensations are related to physiological functions that are in the province of the parasympathetic nervous system.

The autonomic nervous system governs most of our bodily functions—such as respiration, sleep, digestion, heartbeat, and body temperature—and encompasses the sympathetic and parasympathetic networks. The autonomic nervous system maintains homeostasis in the body and is the key to internal stability and balance.

The sympathetic nervous system activates the "fight or flight" response, triggering increased heart rate and blood pressure, sweating, inhibition of digestion, and release of energy stores for use by the large muscle groups. In contrast, the parasympathetic nervous system activates the functions of "rest and digest."

The vagus nerve is part of the parasympathetic nervous system, extending from the medulla in the brain to the base of the spine, forming a network of vital links to the heart, liver, lungs, digestive tract, and other major organs. Most noteworthy about this vital nerve is the correlation between its function and the phenomena people experience when they activate the Water Up, Fire Down energy principle. There is reason to believe that many of these phenomena (including warmth in the abdomen, calming of the heart, teary eyes, and watering mouth) represent increased parasympathetic activity—a rest-and-digest workout for our autonomic nervous system. To those who have experienced a Body & Brain Yoga class, this will sound similar to what happens when they bring their energy down to the dahnjon.

Studies show that many natural health practices, including deep abdominal breathing and acupuncture, can stimulate activity in the parasympathetic nervous system. So the next time you feel energy flowing, remember that you might be helping to improve tone in your autonomic nervous system, too. Although further scientific research is needed, exploring such synergistic effects of energy principle and physiology may forge an expanded understanding of our bodies and minds.

ENERGETIC & PHYSIOLOGICAL
CHANGES WITH WATER UP, FIRE DOWN

[eyes]
Energy flow As water energy reaches the head, the brain is cooled and refreshed; stagnant energy and toxins are released through the mouth (yawns) and eyes (tears).
Parasympathetic activation Stimulation of lacrimal glands releases tears.

[mouth]
Energy flow Circulation of water energy in the head alleviates dry mouth.
Parasympathetic activation Stimulation of mouth glands produces saliva.

[heart]
Energy flow Heat in the heart is cooled as fire energy travels downward toward the abdomen. The mind returns to a stable state.
Parasympathetic activation Slows the heart rate.

[stomach, pancreas]
Energy flow Fire energy travels down to facilitate abdominal organs.
Parasympathetic activation Stomach and pancreas release acids and enzymes that stimulate digestion.

[lungs]
Energy flow Proper breathing, especially with a focus on exhalation, enhances a smooth cycle of descending heat and rising coolness.
Parasympathetic activation Breathing becomes deeper and calmer with less need of oxygen in the body. Constricts airways in the lungs.

[kidneys]
Energy flow Kidneys generate water energy from the fire energy that has gathered in the dahnjon.
Parasympathetic activation Increases blood flow to the kidneys.

[liver]
Energy flow Energy begins to accumulate.
Parasympathetic activation Stimulates the liver for glucose uptake, allowing accumulation of energy stores.

[intestines]
Energy flow Fire energy settles in the lower abdomen and finds its "home" in the dahnjon.
Parasympathetic activation Stimulates contraction of intestinal smooth muscle, promoting absorption of nutrients and flow of bowel contents.

———— Parasympathetic Nerves

THE THREE STEPS TO ENERGY SYSTEM DEVELOPMENT

In Body & Brain Yoga, the natural principles of the energy system are followed to attain health, happiness, and peace. According to these principles, the healthiest way to develop this system begins with the physical body, continues with the energy body, and then completes itself in the spiritual body. This process, also known as the completion of the energy system, develops the three dahnjons from lower to upper. Energy fills the dahnjons from bottom to top, like water poured into a glass, until the whole system is vibrant and filled with pure energy—its most stable and active state. This principle of energy development is called *Jungchoong, Kijang, Shinmyung* in Korean, which translates to "When the body is filled with energy, our energy becomes mature, and our spirituality is awakened." This emphasizes the fulfillment of the lower dahnjon, the physical energy center, as the foundation of the entire energy system. If you want to build a tall building, you need a strong and stable foundation. In the same way, we need a healthy and powerful lower dahnjon to fully develop your energy and spiritual bodies.

Jungchoong: The Body Is Filled with Vital Energy

The physical body is the vessel of earthly life that you received from your parents when you were born into this world. It is sustained by breathing and eating. The lower dahnjon, associated with the physical body, is complete when it is filled with vital energy, or *Jung*, derived from food and air. When you reach the level of Jungchoong (Jung fulfilled), you have fully developed the lower dahnjon, producing an optimal physical condition. You notice an increased adaptability to new surroundings and a resistance to disease. You feel grounded and enjoy physical vitality and stamina. When your Jung is "fulfilled," you can experience the awakening that "My body is not me, but mine." You notice an increased ability to control your energy and channel it according to your will.

Kijang: Energy Becomes Mature

Once your physical body is full of energy, your energy body—ki—begins to mature, meaning that your heart energy becomes clear, full, and strong. The energy body is strongly influenced by your mental and emotional states, which are related to your middle dahnjon. To reach the state of Kijang (mature ki), mental and emotional energy must become light and pure, allowing your heart to open and release the natural wellspring of love and peace within it. Then your middle dahnjon will have completed its development. In the state of Kijang, your mind becomes calm

THE STATE OF JUNGCHOONG, KIJANG, AND SHINMYUNG

Shinmyung
Completion of the upper dahnjon
Enlightenment and spiritual development
Confidence, insight, and totality of being

Kijang
Completion of the middle dahnjon
Mature love, joy, and a sense of peace
Wholeness, compassion, and empathy

Jungchoong
Completion of the lower dahnjon
Optimal physical condition
Enhanced life force

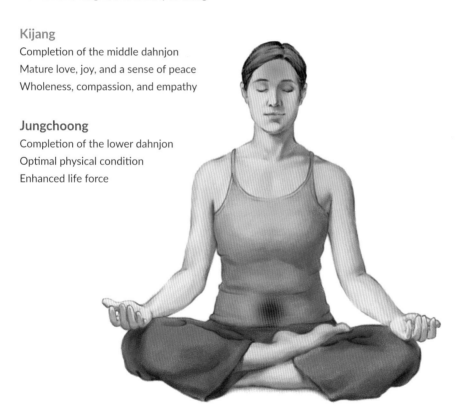

and clear, and your relationships with others and the world become harmonious, peaceful, and boundless. In a sense, Kijang is another way of saying that you are emotionally mature. With the openness and clarity you have gained, you can manage your emotional energy and realize that your emotions and thoughts are not you, but yours to determine.

Shinmyung: Spirituality Is Awakened
Achieving physical and emotional wellness lets you progress to the state of Shinmyung (spirituality awakened)—the completion of the upper dahnjon. At this stage, your consciousness is elevated, achieving total integration of the physical, energy, and spiritual bodies as well as conveying a sense of purpose to life. You develop greater insight, intuition, and judgment, allowing you to sense the essence of a matter without consciously learning about it. Shinmyung lets you use the full power of your body and brain to create your life freely, with a sense of harmony and balance in everything.

FROM MIND TO MATTER
As the foundation of all that exists, energy certainly affects human beings. At the same time, human beings influence energy. Body & Brain Yoga enables you to move and clear energy and use it to create health, happiness, and peace. This ability is based on the principle of *Shim* (mind) *Ki* (energy) *Hyul* (blood) *Jung* (body), which states: "Where consciousness concentrates, energy flows, bringing blood and transforming the body." This principle suggests that consciousness is the true essence of our existence, beyond our physical form. To put Shim Ki Hyul Jung more simply, "Energy goes where the mind goes."

Try this simple exercise to get a better sense of this phenomenon. Breathe in and out a few times to relax your whole body. Concentrate intently on the center of one of your palms. Keep concentrating, and imagine that your palm is becoming hotter than the rest of your body. After a while, you may notice some difference between your two palms. That feeling isn't just "in your head." Real changes occur when you concentrate on your palm, bringing more blood to the area and the warmth that comes with increased circulation.

A keen awareness of energy helps you feel and direct the energy that is moving through your body. Increased sensitivity, along with a greater ability to focus the mind, are natural benefits of Body & Brain Yoga. Through classes and individual practice, you will be able to develop greater power over energy along with an understanding of how to manage it effectively.

The principle of Shim Ki Hyul Jung enables you to align energy and matter with your intention. When you develop the strength and maturity to maintain and protect your intention, you will be able to use the amazing creative power of your mind. You will be able to see your intention, a thought in your consciousness, come into being in the world of form.

For a better understanding of this principle, imagine using a magnifying glass to gather and focus sunlight. If you move the glass around instead of holding it in one place, the sunlight will not accumulate enough power to have any effect. However, if you maintain exact focus in one place for a prolonged period, the energy from the sun will accumulate and create heat. Eventually, enough heat will build up to create fire. In just the same way, our thoughts are powerful when focused on a single intention or goal; they're capable of generating life-changing phenomena.

The principle of Shim Ki Hyul Jung provides profound insight into living a more creative life. When consciousness becomes concentrated, energy gathers. This in turn begins to attract the materials necessary to manifest the essence of the concentrated consciousness. Hyul, which literally means "blood," actually refers to all the material components required to generate the physical form of an intention. Thus, Shim Ki Hyul Jung refers to the process of invisible consciousness creating tangible forms through the power of concentration. This is related to what some call the "Law of Attraction."

The unity of consciousness, energy, and physical matter that underlies Shim Ki Hyul Jung has been dubbed by Ilchi Lee as "LifeParticles"—the smallest units of life. It is the unified nature of LifeParticles that makes Shim Ki Hyul Jung possible and allows thoughts to manifest themselves in the physical world. The universe is filled with LifeParticles that we can draw on to turn our innermost dreams and visions, whatever they may be, into reality.

Three Main Methods of Energy Practice

Body & Brain Yoga achieves the development and healthy functioning of the body's energy system through three main methods of practice—*Jigam* (stop emotion), *Joshik* (control breathing), and *Geumchok* (detach from stimulation). Jigam quiets your thoughts and emotions, Joshik governs your mind by regulating your energy through breathing, and Geumchok frees you from the external stimuli disturbing your center. Using the body and mind's natural tendencies, these practices help restore balance and clear away confusion to reveal our center, our true self. They also strengthen the power of the mind to the point where we can choose the thoughts and emotions that align with our goals. The final destination of all these practices is full connection with your true self.

When we don't have Water Up, Fire Down energy circulation and our lower dahnjon isn't strong enough, our thoughts may pull us in one direction while our emotions pull us in another, and our physical needs may tug us on a completely different path. The chronic stress and hectic pace of the typical modern lifestyle keep our minds constantly stimulated and focused on the external world. The noise within us becomes as great as the noise around us. Our brain waves and nervous system remain in an overactive and even agitated state. In this condition, it's difficult to focus energy and be able to accumulate adequate pure energy in the body. It's also difficult to maintain awareness of our true self and what it wants.

Without awareness, the thoughts and emotions that make up our inner world tend to pull us in whatever direction our habits prefer, trapping us in our comfort zone and pulling us in a direction we may not want to go. Jigam, Joshik, and Geumchok help us see our patterns clearly and separate our awareness from the chorus of thoughts and emotions. Given more space and awareness, we are better able to change the habits of both body and brain.

JIGAM: STOP EMOTION

Jigam literally translates as "stop emotion." It means having a clear, calm mind that is free of emotional agitation. Have your emotions ever stopped? Emotions fluctuate almost constantly in our lives. Particularly when negative thoughts and feelings arise, we experience conflicts, distress, and distracting thoughts that consume vital energy. This keeps us from accumulating energy, weakening the body and mind and causing us to suffer from all kinds of illnesses.

However, thoughts and emotions can be stilled through meditation, which centers the mind. When we focus on just one thing, the mind naturally becomes calmer and emotions tend to diminish. This isn't easy, especially when we're just trying to control our thoughts. Try too hard, and the noise inside actually grows louder. That's why Body & Brain Yoga practice uses physical stimulation to capture the mind's attention. The mind has a natural propensity to pay attention to physical sensations in order to protect us. Our thoughts and emotions become more stable when we focus on our physical sensations.

In Jigam, the physical sensation we concentrate on is the feeling of the body's energy. When we feel the ceaseless circulation of energy in and out of and through the body, our brain wave frequency slows to below an alpha level and our thoughts and feelings calm down. We can enter a state of serenity, and more energy can accumulate in the body. As a form of meditation, focusing on the energy flowing through the body doesn't require a lot of practice. Even if feeling energy seems difficult in the beginning, the effort of focusing will begin to help quiet emotions and thoughts.

Of all the parts of the body, the hands are especially sensitive to sensation. They are filled with nerve endings, and many brain structures are assigned to process signals from the hands. For most people, the hands are the first place they feel energy. As we feel energy flow into and between our palms, our minds stay in the present moment instead of roaming to past memories or future plans. Our brain waves slow to a meditative state and our bodies go into "rest and digest" mode. Jigam with our hands stimulates the Jangshim energy points in the palms, releasing emotions built up in the chest and letting fresh energy fill the middle dahnjon. The fire energy in the chest and the head will then flow down more easily to the lower dahnjon, facilitating Water Up, Fire Down energy flow.

The heart opening and energy expansion we experience through Jigam brings true peace, and a smile to the face. Eventually, the sensation of energy will expand beyond our palms to the whole body. Immersed in the here and now, we can feel our sense of self expand beyond the limits of the physical body, and we may feel connected to everything and everyone around us. After creating this quiet, focused state, we can turn our attention to our true self in our heart and listen to its dreams and wisdom. We can see what's missing in our lives, and be grateful for what is there. Jigam allows us experience ourselves at the deepest level.

For detailed instructions on how to practice Jigam, see Chapter 6, page 101.

JOSHIK: CONTROL BREATHING

Joshik means "control breathing." Breathing is one of the few vital processes that we can control. Through breathing, we can manage our minds, emotions, and energy.

We breathe unconsciously all the time, but we can control our breathing by consciously paying attention to our breath. As you will see later in this book, Body &

Brain Yoga breathing exercises consist of breathing in different postures. Simply by bringing our awareness to our breath, our breathing will begin to slow and deepen. Slow and deep breathing in which the abdomen rises and falls calms the mind and relaxes the body.

Abdominal breathing in a relaxed state lets energy accumulate in the body, particularly in the lower dahnjon. With each breath, we inhale fresh energy and exhale stagnant energy. By controlling breath, we can control energy flow, gathering energy to activate and refresh the entire energy system. The deeper our breathing, the more energy we take in. A Water Up, Fire Down energy state can be naturally created and Jungchoong, Kijang, Shinmyung achieved. By intentionally controlling our energy state through breathing, we not only calm our thoughts and emotions but are able to purposely direct them and imbue them with vitality and positivity.

Breathing, of course, is essential to life. It is an expression of life. When we breathe with devotion, we can become one with the natural rhythm of life and experience the preciousness of our own lives. In the state of deep awareness that we can enter through Joshik, we are able to experience becoming one with the universe when we exhale and one with the body when we inhale. The boundary between inside and outside slips away. We realize that the substance of who we are isn't bound by anything. It stays neither inside nor outside; it exists everywhere in every moment.

Breathing is something we all do from the moment we are born, even without learning how. Once we know its true meaning, though, we can understand this simple yet deep level of training. Through breathing alone, we can become the true masters of our bodies and minds, by unifying the comings and goings of breath and energy and then circulating energy with the power of the mind.

There are many breathing exercises practiced in Body & Brain Yoga, and breathing is a part of every class. The basic breathing exercises are found in Chapter 6, pages 124–140.

GEUMCHOK: DETACH FROM STIMULATION

Geumchok means "detach from stimulation." Geumchok is a cutting ourselves off from outside information entering through our five sensory organs—eyes, ears, nose, tongue, and skin—and focusing our awareness on a place deep within. We encounter the fundamental substance of life inside ourselves when we break sensory communication with the external world and our consciousness focuses entirely within.

Geumchok is most effective when practiced in daily life as well as in formal training. Put simply, it's about distancing yourself as much as possible from whatever disturbs your inner center. For this, you shouldn't be overly attached to things you love or to things you hate. Driven by such likes and dislikes, it's easy to lose your center. For example, if you tend to indulge in food, alcohol, or tobacco, you're being led about by the external—by sensory things. In addition to such physical factors, the feelings and thoughts arising from personal relationships and external information are also stimuli that disrupt your center. To begin your practice, intentionally distance yourself from such stimuli. Later, when your center is firmly established, such stimuli won't even phase you; you'll have reached a level where you can be free of them. This is the real state of Geumchok.

Body & Brain Yoga offers methods for easily entering the state of Geumchok. One example is Yeondahn, in which you hold a single posture for a long time, are Geumchok on an active level for strengthening your core. The most common Yeondahn posture is called Sleeping Tiger. You can find instructions for doing Sleeping Tiger in Chapter 6 on pages 134–135.

Signs of Healing

THE VIBRATION OF LIFE

Many changes occur in the body during Body & Brain Yoga exercises, differing from one person to the next. Without some understanding of what is happening to the body as a result of the energy stimulation that takes place, some people might feel frightened or confused when they experience these changes.

One sign that the body is changing is that it begins to move spontaneously. This reaction is the result of moving into a deeply relaxed, alpha brain wave state. As a person begins to feel the flow of energy circulating throughout the body, the body may stretch deeply on its own, shake minutely or violently, or jerk suddenly as blockages in the meridians are cleared by the flood of energy. This can be compared to suddenly turning the water on full blast on a garden hose. With the increase in water pressure, the hose begins to shake and move around. Likewise, the body will vibrate when energy suddenly begins to flow.

There are two types of vibration. In one case, vibration occurs when suffi-cient energy accumulates in the dahnjon that it begins to flow rapidly through the meridian system. In the second case, vibration can result from an influx of vital cosmic energy after the mind is fully opened.

Practitioners with good energy circulation may not experience vibration at first. But as their training deepens, most practitioners experience the vibration of life. Or some practitioners may not sense the vibration because it is so delicate.

Vibration is a sign that Body & Brain Yoga practice is having an effect, and a person's health will improve after such an experience. Most people feel refreshed after experiencing vibration, since blocked meridian channels have been opened. The mind feels steady and strong, and physical health improves dramatically.

MYUNGHYUN: ALTERNATING BRIGHTNESS AND DARKNESS

Nature is cyclical. Day turns to night, and night turns to day. The body's energy system is a climate, too, continuously fluctuating between dark and light. Body & Brain Yoga exercises increase and free energy, making the system lighter and brighter as heavier energy is released. In the process, toxins held by stagnant energy are washed out of the body.

As the energy system begins to release stagnant energies, uncomfortable sensations, called Myunghyun, may appear. Myunghyun literally translates as "brightness" (myung) and "darkness" (hyun). Symptoms persist until energy is able to flow freely. Although Myunghyun may feel uncomfortable, its symptoms indicate that the body is restoring itself.

Myunghyun phenomena may include both physical and emotional symptoms. Practitioners may feel unexplained levels of fatigue or have flu-like symptoms. After the symptoms disappear, energy levels increase. Bruise-like stains may appear on the skin at the sites of old injuries, or an old pain may return briefly. Similarly, there may be a recurrence of a health problem or an unusual physical sensation, such as a persistent vibration in some part of the body. Strong waves of cold or heat could suddenly emanate from the center of the body. Such symptoms indicate that healing has started to occur at the energy level, not just at a physiological level. Physical Myunghyun symptoms are alleviated when the body's basic energy flow is optimized to the state of Water Up, Fire Down.

Myunghyun phenomena can also occur when old emotional habits begin to change and negative emotional energies are released. Emotional Myunghyun can be manifested as inexplicable mood swings, sudden depression, or angry outbursts.

When you experience Myunghyun, remain positive and grateful for the opportunity to become more energetic. Where your mind goes, energy follows. If your mind is bright and positive, bright and positive energy will come to you.

If you experience Myunghyun, you may feel that you don't want to continue your practice. However, maintaining your practice is usually the most efficient way to recover. If you are going to a Body & Brain Yoga Center, consult your instructor about your experience.

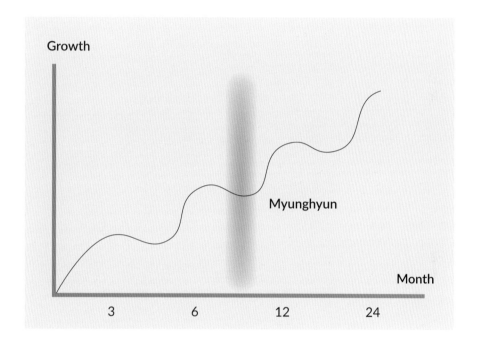

Progress of Practice

PART 2
THE PRACTICE

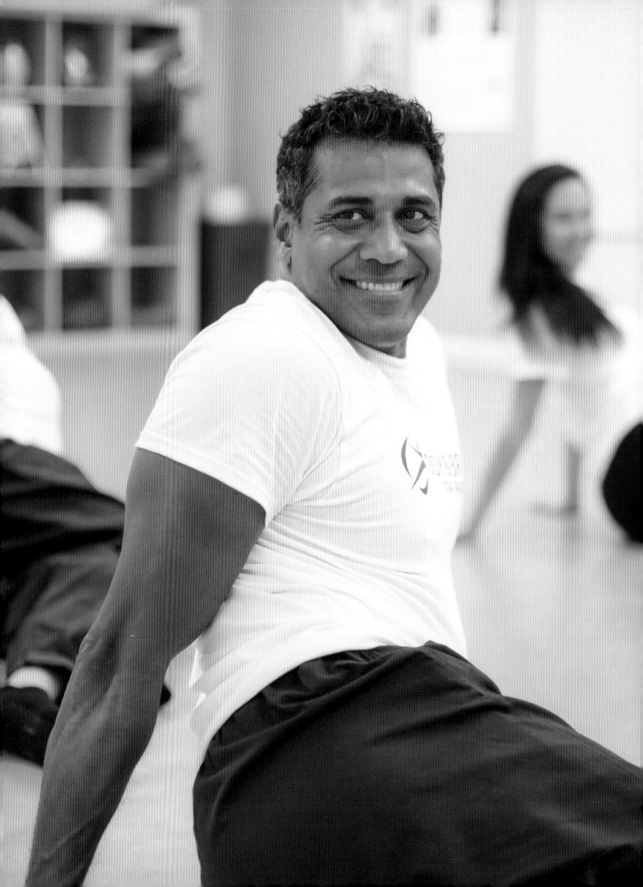

CHAPTER 6

BODY & BRAIN YOGA IN PRACTICE

The Components of Body & Brain Yoga

Body & Brain Yoga programs consist of seven major components designed to achieve the optimal energy conditions for body and brain. Each of these can be an effective training method when done independently, but the best results are achieved if all are performed together over a daily training session of an hour to an hour and a half.

WARM-UP EXERCISES

The degree to which you'll benefit from Body & Brain Yoga exercises depends on the strength of your lower dahnjon. As discussed earlier in relation to the principle of Jungchoong Kijang Shinmyung, a strong dahnjon is not only a source of physical power and resilience but also a foundation of emotional wellness and maturity as well as mental clarity and creativity. Warm-up exercises consist of movements that create the Water Up, Fire Down energy balance quickly and effectively by bringing the energy in the head to the lower dahnjon.

MERIDIAN EXERCISES

These deep stretching, twisting, and joint rotation movements can help improve circulation and body alignment. When combined with mindful breathing and body awareness, they stimulate energy circulation through the body's energy pathways, or meridians. When circulation is blocked and stagnant, the body's energy sensation becomes dull. Meridian Exercises help facilitate energy circulation by relaxing the body, eliminating stagnant energy, and supplying fresh energy.

RELAXATION

Body & Brain Yoga mainly uses the body's energy sensation and visualization for relaxation, along with signature exercises that have powerful relaxation effects, such as Brain Wave Vibration and Belly Button Healing. Through these practices you learn to shift your focus away from busy thoughts through enhanced energy awareness. When you are relaxed, you can more deeply experience the benefits of breathing and meditation.

BREATHING

Body & Brain Yoga's breathing exercises help build energy in the lower dahnjon and unblock meridians, especially the Conception Vessel meridian and the Governing Vessel meridian running along the body's midline. These exercises consist of natural breathing in specific postures, which helps to restore Water Up, Fire Down energy circulation. Consistent practice can improve energy accumulation and circulation and stimulate the body's natural healing ability.

MEDITATION

To achieve a meditative state, Body & Brain Yoga mainly uses energy meditation and moving meditation combined with breathing. Both increase energy flow and awareness. While increased sensitivity to energy is a definite benefit of this practice, it is not the end goal. Rather, the aim is to calm thoughts and emotions—the root cause of stress held in the body. Once body and mind become more relaxed, practitioners learn to recreate their lives through vision meditation, which infuses the mind with positive thoughts, feelings, and imagery.

KIGONG AND TAI CHI

Some Body & Brain Yoga classes include kigong exercises and tai chi forms to strengthen the ability to sense and use energy. These forms also strengthen lower body muscles and dahnjon energy. The specific postures and movements that are used help loosen joints and realign bone structure. The movements can be strong or gentle, but all are designed to create harmony of body and mind.

WRAP-UP EXERCISES

These movements energize body and mind after being in a state of deep relaxation with stabilized brain waves. They are usually gentle Meridian Exercises that are good for lengthening muscles, rejuvenating energy, refocusing on the core, and creating circulation in the entire body.

Body & Brain Yoga in Practice

WARM-UP EXERCISES

Each Body & Brain Yoga class typically begins with one or more exercises to warm up the body. Mainly composed of movements to strengthen the dahnjon in the lower abdomen, these warm-up exercises bring the energy in the head down to the dahnjon. Within the abdomen are digestive organs, circulatory organs, immune organs, and other major organs necessary to maintain life. Exercises that stimulate the lower abdomen not only help blood and energy circulate in the abdomen, but they also improve digestion and detoxify and activate the metabolism. The gut is particularly sensitive to stress and also directly affects brain function. Warm-up exercises are effective for relaxing the intestines and the gut overall, helping to relieve stress. They also make the dahnjon feel warm, which means that its energy sense has been activated.

DAHNJON TAPPING

BENEFITS: Dahnjon Tapping is a simple but effective way to strengthen the lower abdomen, especially the dahnjon. By rhythmically patting the lower abdomen with the palms of both hands, you distribute blood and energy throughout your entire body. Abdominal exercises such as this assist in the prompt removal of excess gases and waste, and they increase the feeling of warmth in the dahnjon.

NOTE: *Begin with 100 taps. You can increase the number and strength with more practice.*

1. Spread your feet shoulder-width apart and bend your knees slightly.

2. Lengthen and relax your spine. Relax your shoulders, neck, and arms.

3. Point your toes slightly inward so that the outer sides of your feet are parallel and you feel a slight tightening of the lower abdomen.

4. Rhythmically tap the lower abdomen area with both palms, keeping your arms loose.

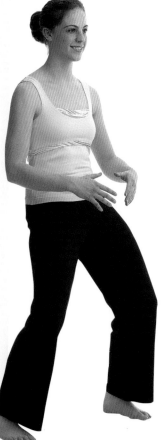
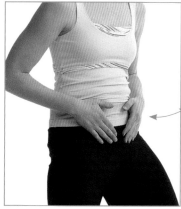

INTESTINAL EXERCISE

BENEFITS: This exercise increases the flexibility of the intestines and facilitates efficient circulation of energy and blood. If you tighten your rectal muscles while doing the exercise, you'll be able to gather energy and feel warmth much more quickly.

NOTE: *Don't overdo this exercise in the beginning, or it may cause some discomfort. Start with one set of 50 and work your way up to a set of 300 as you advance.*

This exercise can be performed standing up, sitting, or lying down in many different positions. The basic position is the same as for Dahnjon Tapping—standing with feet shoulder-width apart, knees slightly bent, toes turned slightly inward. If sitting, use a half lotus posture or sit in a chair with both feet parallel on the ground; keep your spine straight. If lying down, lie on your back with your feet shoulder-width apart.

1. Whichever posture you use, form a triangle with your hands by touching your thumbs and fore-fingers together. Place your hands lightly on your lower abdomen so that your thumbs meet over your navel.

2. Pull in the front wall of your abdomen, as if it were trying to touch your back. Tighten your rectal muscles at the same time.

3. Now push your lower abdomen out slightly, making it more rounded. You will feel outward pressure in your lower abdomen.

4. Repeat the movement.

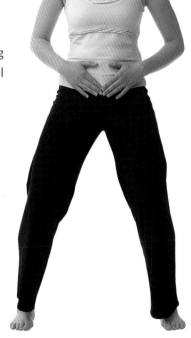

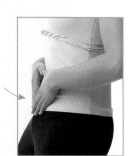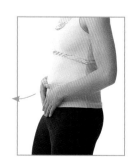

MERIDIAN EXERCISES

Meridian Exercises are designed to unblock stuck energy in the body's energy channels, put the body back into alignment, and relax both body and mind. In these exercises, breathing and focusing the mind are combined with stretching, rotating, shaking, and squeezing movements that target different meridians. When breath is combined with body movement, metabolism is more effectively influenced.

There are hundreds of Meridian Exercises. This book introduces a sampling of the most effective ones for relaxing the body and circulating energy. They let the concentration of energy come down into the lower dahnjon and limber up the pelvis (which is like a bowl that collects the energy) and the hip joints (which are like energy faucets).

Although Meridian Exercises are used primarily before and after breathing and meditation, practicing them on their own greatly helps to maintain health and prevent illness.

RELAXING THE UPPER BODY
Breathing and meditation can't be fully experienced when tension is held in the upper body. When the shoulders and chest are blocked in this way, energy stagnates in the upper body instead of gathering in the dahnjon. Then the healthy state of Water Up, Fire Down is reversed. Meridian Exercises focus on relaxing the upper body while drawing the energy down into the lower dahnjon.

MAKING THE HIP JOINTS NIMBLE
Meridian Exercises include various movements to make the hip joints flexible and strong. Training the muscles around the hip joints makes energy circulation and blood flow smoother while helping the accumulated energy in the dahnjon spread throughout the body.

HARMONIZING MOVEMENT, BREATHING, AND AWARENESS
To optimize the effects of Meridian Exercises, movement, breathing, and awareness must be harmonized. Start the movements while inhaling. Hold your breath for a moment while holding the posture called for, then exhale slowly while returning to the beginning position. Your body should be centered at the lower dahnjon, and your consciousness should be focused on the areas being stretched. When

exhaling, imagine that the stagnating energy in the body is leaving. Imagine that you are having a conversation with your body and focus on the changes or sensations that you feel.

It's important to practice Meridian Exercises in a way that is suitable for your body. For example, a healthy and flexible person can train more intensely, whereas a weaker and less flexible person can practice the movements more gently. Even ill and fragile individuals can benefit from gently rubbing and massaging the whole body while breathing and focusing their awareness on the body. In the beginning, work on mastering the movements rather than attempting to harmonize breathing and movements. When you are familiar with the movements, practice them according to your own breathing capacity, without straining.

Standing Meridian Exercises

THE BASIC POSTURE

SHOULDERS Relax your shoulders.

WAIST Straighten your waist and curl in the tailbone, like a hook. This straightens the S-curve of the spine and puts a gentle strain on the lower abdomen.

KNEES Bend your knees slightly and naturally. Avoid locking them, since this can block energy flow.

LEGS Spread your legs so that your feet are shoulder-width apart but no more than that. Spreading them too far apart can scatter the energy of the dahnjon and lower body.

FEET Position your feet parallel to each other, like the number 11. Balance your weight evenly on both feet.

BREATHING Inhale gently through the nose, imagining healing energy flowing to whatever part of the body feels tense or painful. Open your mouth slightly, exhale naturally, and feel the blockage being released from your body.

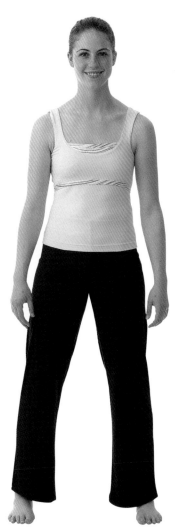

BODY BOUNCE

BENEFITS: This exercise helps reduce tension and release stagnant energy from the whole body. It also enhances blood and energy circulation and loosens joints.

NOTE: *Breathe naturally while rhythmically bouncing your whole body up and down.*

1. Stand with your feet shoulder-width apart.

2. Bend your knees slightly and begin to bounce your body gently.

3. As you rhythmically bounce your entire body up and down, sweep the sides of your body with your fingertips about 10 times.

4. Continue this movement as you turn your body 45 degrees to the left without moving your feet and rhythmically bounce and sweep 10 times.

5. Now turn 45 degrees to the right and rhythmically bounce your body up and down while sweeping your hands down your body another 10 times.

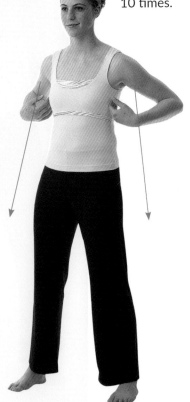

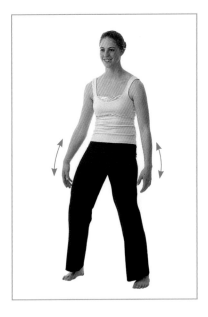

UPPER BODY TAPPING

BENEFITS: This exercise helps energy circulation, opens energy blockages, and releases stagnant energy from the whole body. It enhances blood circulation and relaxes the chest and abdominal area.

NOTE: *If you feel discomfort in any area that you are tapping, tap more lightly. This is particularly important if you experience stomach distress. Also, don't press into the area where you feel discomfort. Instead, gently rub your hands together and then lightly rub the area.*

1. Stand with your feet shoulder-width apart and parallel to each other. Relax your upper body, bend your knees slightly, and balance your weight evenly on both feet.

2. Make light fists and gently tap your chest, stomach, ribs, and entire abdominal area while exhaling with an "Aaah" sound.

3. Continue tapping for 5 minutes.

4. Focus your awareness on the places where you feel achy and stiff, then breathe out with the feeling of releasing the impure energy accumulated in those areas.

5. Close your eyes and focus on the vibration of the tapping as it penetrates deep inside the body.

WHOLE BODY PATTING

BENEFITS: This is an effective method for reducing tension and releasing energy from your whole body. By patting, you open energy points.

NOTE: *Pat the body gently and comfortably to achieve the desired results. You'll be able to concentrate better if you follow your movements with your eyes.*

1. Stand with your feet shoulder-width apart and your knees slightly bent.

2. Curl your fingers and use your fingertips to tap lightly all over your head and face.

3. Stretch your left arm out in front of you, palm facing up. With your right hand, start at the left shoulder and rhythmically pat down the left arm all the way to the hand.

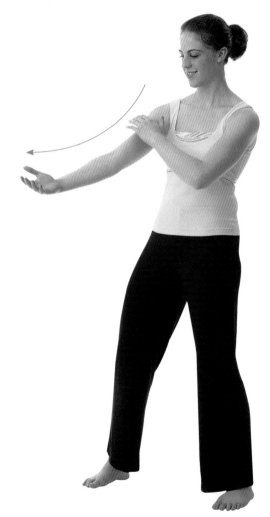

4. Then turn your left hand palm down and use your right hand to pat your way back up to the left shoulder.

5. Repeat Steps 2 and 3 with the right arm out and the left hand patting it.

6. Pat your chest several times with both hands, exhaling completely.

7. Now pat the front and sides of your ribs.

8. Using both hands, pat the area just below the left rib cage where your stomach is located. Concentrate on bringing healing energy to your stomach.

9. Using both hands, pat the area just below the right rib cage where your liver is located. Concentrate on radiating positive, clear energy to the liver.

10. Bend over slightly from the waist and reach back to pat the area on your lower back (both sides) where your kidneys are located.

11. Now move up the back, patting as far as you can reach. Then pat your way down to your buttocks.

12. Starting from your buttocks, pat your way down the backs of your legs to your ankles.

13. From the ankles, start patting up the front of your legs from the top of your feet to the front of your hips.

14. From the sides of your hips, pat your way down the outsides of your legs to your ankles.

15. From your insteps, pat your way up the insides of your legs.

16. Finish by tapping your lower abdomen about 20 times.

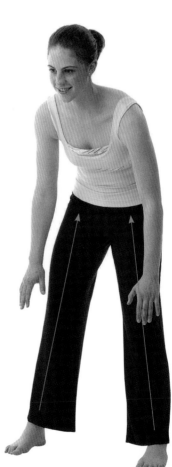

PLATE BALANCING

BENEFITS: This full-body exercise loosens all of the joints in the body, particularly in the back and shoulders. It also aids balance and coordination and stimulates energy, blood, and lymph circulation throughout the body. When time is limited, doing Plate Balancing on its own—even several times a day—keeps the body warm, strong, balanced, and limber.

NOTE: *If you don't have a plate available, use another object or just imagine that you're holding one. Follow the hand(s) holding the plate with your eyes for the greatest benefit. Do each set of movements 10 times or more.*

WITH ONE HAND

1. Plant your right foot forward from the other foot by about one and a half times your shoulder width, toes pointing forward. Turn the left foot outward at about a 45-degree angle. Bend your knees slightly. Your stance should feel comfortable, balanced, and natural. Balance a plate on the palm of your right hand and hold it at elbow height over your right knee. Rest the back of your left hand against your back.

2. While leaning your upper body forward, pull your right hand—with the plate balanced on it—in toward your body in a counterclockwise circle, pivoting around your elbow until your arm is straight out to the side and twisted so that your palm is still facing upward. With your elbow straight, continue the circle by moving your shoulder until your arm is extended in front of you. Keep your palm facing up.

3. Begin a second circle by moving your arm counter-clockwise over your head as you extend your upper body back as far as you can and straighten your right (front) knee while bending your left (back) knee. Look back at your hand as it circles behind you. Twist your arm as much as you need to in order to keep your palm (and your plate) facing upward. As your hand passes behind you and comes around to its original position in front of you, straighten your upper body.

4. Repeat this spiraling motion several times, then reverse the direction and spiral the plate in a clockwise direction.

5. Now switch the position of your feet and repeat the sequence with the plate balanced on your left hand.

Start Here

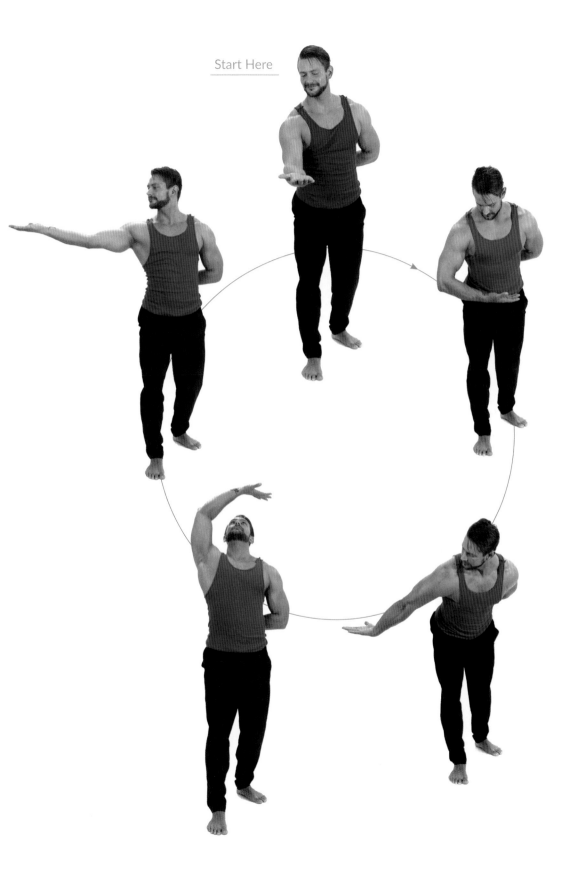

WITH BOTH HANDS

1. Standing with your feet close together and your palms facing up, bend your elbows about 90 degrees and hold your elbows comfortably by your waist. If you have difficulty keeping your balance in this position, place your feet about shoulder-width apart. Balance a plate on each palm, or you may choose not to use plates. You can also hold the plates in place with your thumbs.

2. Bend your upper body forward, bringing your hips back and straightening your knees as much as you can. Keeping your knees straight will provide the most benefit to your back and legs. However, if you have trouble balancing in this position, you can bend your knees.

3. As you bend forward, slowly pivot your hands around your elbows in toward your body until your arms are out to the sides. With your palms facing up, continue the circle until your arms are extended out in front of you.

4. Straighten your upper body, crossing your arms in front of you as you raise up.

5. Now lean your upper body backward as you move each hand above your head in the biggest circle you can make out to the sides, until your hands come back to their original positions.

Start Here

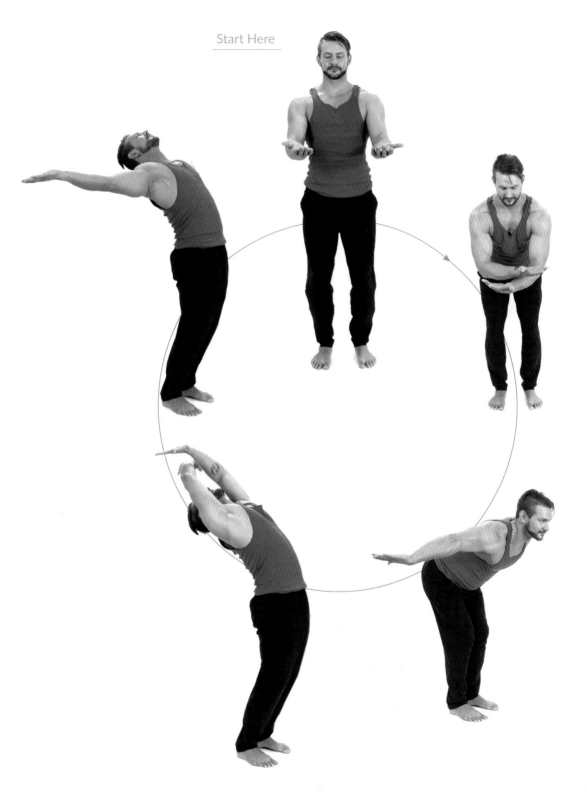

NECK STRETCH

BENEFITS: This stretch eases tension, increases flexibility, and tones the neck muscles. If your neck starts to feel tight in the middle of the working day, this is a simple way to release muscle tension.

NOTE: *Maintain focus on your neck as you perform these movements. Move only your neck and head, very slowly. Relax the rest of your body.*

1. Breathe in and push your chin slowly down to your chest. Exhale and bring your neck back up.

2. Breathe in and stretch your neck backward. Feel your chin and neck stretch. Exhale and bring your neck back to the original position.

3. Breathe in and bend your head sideways to the left, trying to touch your left ear to your shoulder. Exhale and bring your neck back up.

4. Repeat the movement in the opposite direction, bending your head to the right.

5. Breathe in and slowly turn your head to the left. Exhale and turn your head forward again.

6. Repeat the movement in the opposite direction, turning your head to the right.

7. Now rotate your head counterclockwise. Inhale as your head goes back, then exhale it comes forward. Repeat 3 times.

8. Do Step 7 in the opposite direction 3 times.

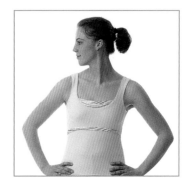

SHOULDER ROTATION

BENEFITS: This exercise helps to open up and tone tight shoulder and upper back muscles.

NOTE: *You don't need to try to make the circles too big. Your joints shouldn't click or feel strained, and your shoulders shouldn't hunch. Imagine that you are oiling the insides of the shoulder joints.*

1. Rest your hands lightly on your shoulders.

2. Inhale and lift your elbows to your sides at shoulder height.

3. Slowly rotate your shoulders back, making large circles with your elbows. Repeat 10 times.

4. Then rotate forward 10 times.

5. Exhale as you bring your elbows back down.

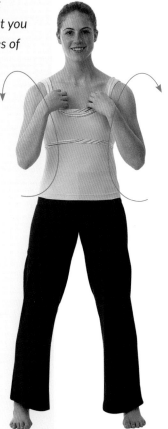

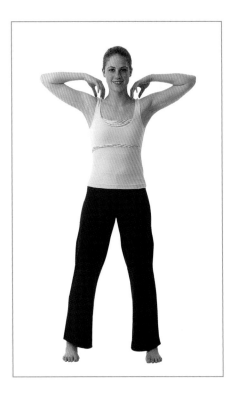

ARM TWISTS

BENEFITS: These movements facilitate the flow of energy by loosening muscles and joints. They also help to release arm and shoulder stiffness.

NOTE: *This motion is like wringing the water out of a towel.*

1. Stand with your feet shoulder-width apart. Raise your arms out to your sides, level with your shoulders, palms down.

2. Breathing in, twist both arms forward as far as they will go. Breathe out as you return to your starting position.

3. Breathing in, twist both arms backward as far as they will go. Breathe out as you return to your starting position.

4. Breathing in, twist both arms in a clockwise direction as far as they will go, keeping your eyes on the right arm. Your right arm twists backward, your left arm forward. Relax while breathing out and returning to the starting position.

5. Breathing in, twist both arms in a counterclockwise direction as far as they will go, keeping your eyes on the left arm. Your left arm twists backward, your right arm forward. Relax while breathing out and returning to the starting position.

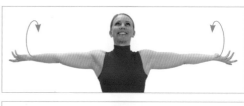

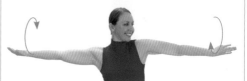

CHEST OPENING

BENEFITS: Stress, tension, and fire energy are released from the chest and shoulders, allowing energy to circulate to the lower dahnjon. This also facilitates deeper breathing.

NOTE: *This exercise can be performed standing or sitting. Release the stagnant energy in your chest by exhaling through the mouth with each motion.*

1. If standing, have your feet parallel and shoulder-width apart and your knees slightly bent. If sitting, sit up straight in a chair, away from the chair back, with your feet flat on the ground, or sit on the floor in a half lotus posture.

2. Raise your arms out to your sides at shoulder height, with your elbows bent and your forearms raised up at 90 degrees, your fists up in the air.

3. With your head facing forward, twist your torso back and forth to each side, keeping your elbows in a straight line with your shoulders and each other. Do this 10 times, focusing on the center of your chest as you move.

4. Now rest your fingertips lightly on your shoulders while keeping your elbows straight out to your sides at shoulder height. Facing forward, bend from one side to the other, keeping your elbows raised. Bend to each side 10 times. Focus your mind on the sides of your rib cage.

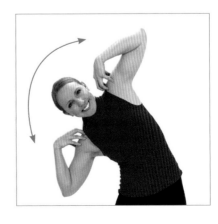

STANDING STRETCH

BENEFITS: This exercise stimulates the meridians on the sides and the back of the body and enhances blood circulation to the heart. It stretches the arm and shoulder muscles and optimizes the function of the liver and other organs.

NOTE: *Breathe deeply in each position, and let yourself stretch a little farther with each inhalation.*

1. Put your feet together and clasp your fingers together in front of you.

2. Breathing in, lift your clasped hands above your head, palms facing the sky, until your arms are touching your ears on either side.

3. At the same time, lift your heels and tilt your head backward to look at your hands.

4. Now lower your feet and hands slowly as you breathe out.

5. Again, stretch your arms upward, palms facing up. Inhale and tilt your whole body to the right as far as you can without losing your balance. Hold your breath for 3 seconds as you feel your whole left side being stretched.

6. Return to an upright position and lower your hands as you breathe out.

7. Repeat the same motion to the left. Feel your whole right side being stretched.

8. Return to an upright position and lower your hands as you breathe out.

9. Now breathe in as you bend forward from the waist and try to touch the ground with your clasped hands, palms down. Be careful not to bend your knees. Try to touch your knees with your forehead, or come as close as you can.

10. Return to the starting position as you exhale.

11. Repeat the whole cycle 3 times.

Start Here

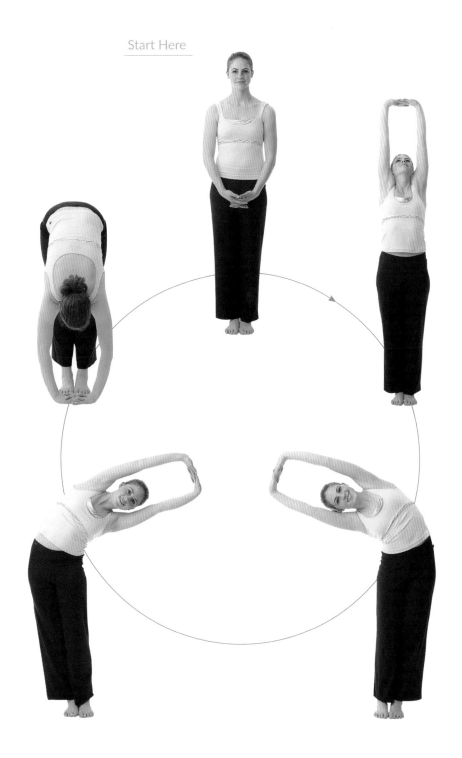

HIP ROTATION

BENEFITS: This exercise helps strengthen the hips, buttocks, and hamstrings.

NOTE: *As you do these exercises, it is most important to feel the hip joints, sacrum, and area surrounding them, including your thighs.*

1. Relax your upper body and gently curl up your tailbone while standing straight to create firm but gentle tension in the lower abdomen.

2. With your hands lightly clasped behind your back and your feet a couple of inches apart, lift the right knee up to the lower dahnjon level and rotate your hip outward 10 times.

3. Relax your chest as you rotate, while trying to keep your right foot from touching the ground.

4. Switch legs and repeat the same motion 10 times with the left knee and hip.

5. Lift the right knee again and rotate it 10 times in the opposite direction.

6. Change legs and repeat the same motion 10 times with the left knee.

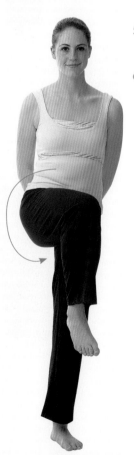

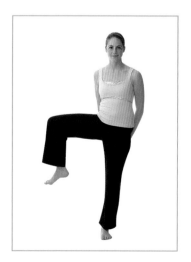

PELVIC ROTATION

BENEFITS: This exercise will train the muscles in your waist, buttocks, hip, thighs, and legs.

NOTE: *Relax your chest and rotate your pelvis while keeping your upper body straight.*

1. Stand with your feet as far apart as possible so that the ligaments in the hip joint can be stretched. Bend your knees slightly and make your spine straight from the tailbone to the top of the neck.

2. Rotate your pelvis and hips from left to right 10 times. Concentrate on the sensation of the pelvic movement and on your exhalation. Keep your knees and chest stationary.

3. Now reverse direction, rotating from right to left 10 times.

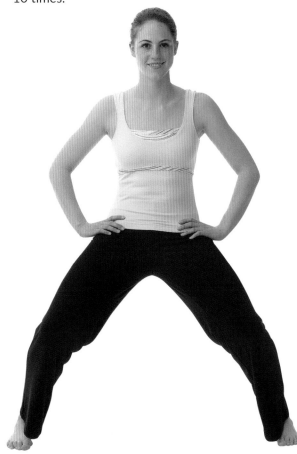

KNEE ROTATION

BENEFITS: This exercise promotes optimal blood and energy circulation in the knee joints and helps relieve knee pain.

NOTE: *While you are rotating your knees, don't let the bottoms of your feet lift off the ground. Don't put any weight on your knees with your hands. Relax your upper body fully and let your weight rest only below the knees.*

1. Standing with knees together, bend your upper body forward and massage your knees and kneecaps with your hands.

2. Slightly bend your knees and keep your feet flat on the floor. Lightly place a hand on each knee.

3. Keep your knees together as you rotate them in a circular motion toward the right 10 times.

4. Repeat the same movement 10 times in the opposite direction.

5. Now rotate your knees from inside to outside 10 times.

6. Repeat the same movement 10 times in the opposite direction.

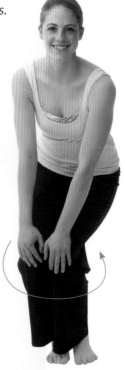

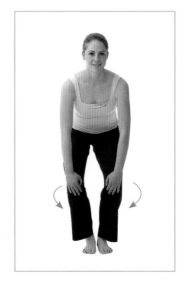

Sitting & Lying Down Meridian Exercises

SITTING FORWARD BEND

BENEFITS: This exercise opens the meridians on the back side of the body and stretches the entire body, from the heels to the top of the spine.

NOTE: *Aim to bring your torso as far down as possible while keeping knees and spine straight. If you focus on bringing your head to your legs, neglecting your torso, this will curve your spine.*

1. Sit on the floor with your legs together, stretching them straight out in front of you.

2. Inhale and bring your arms out to the sides and up over your head.

3. Bend your torso forward, keeping your lower back straight. Lower your arms as you do this so that your hands can touch your toes. Try to pull your toes toward your body and keep your legs straight. Bend at the elbow as you bring your chest and head toward your knees.

4. Exhale and return to your original posture.

5. Repeat several times.

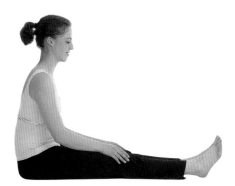

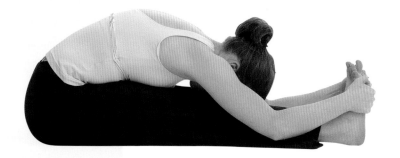

STRADDLE WITH FORWARD BEND

MERIDIAN EXERCISES

BENEFITS: This exercise stretches and lengthens the natural curve of the spine, hip joints, and hamstrings. It squeezes the abdominal organs and nourishes them with fresh blood and energy.

NOTE: *Avoid over-stretching your thighs by taking most of your weight on your hands at first. Little by little, inch your way forward until you can bring your elbows down.*

1. Sit on the floor and stretch your legs apart as far as you can. Point your toes upward.

2. Put your palms on the floor in front of you with your fingers facing each other. Bounce your upper body forward several times, bending your elbows as you do so.

3. After bouncing, reach your hands toward your ankles, trying to touch them as you bend your upper torso toward the ground. Try to bring your chest and chin all the way to the floor while keeping your spine straight.

4. Repeat several times.

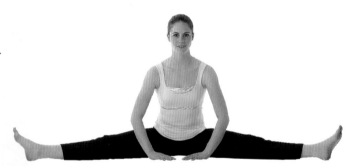

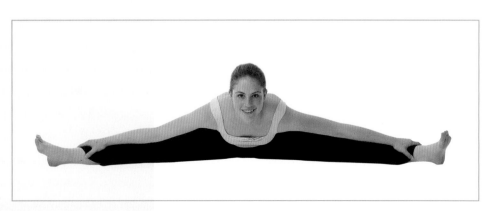

SIDE STRETCH

BENEFITS: This exercise gives an excellent stretch to the spine, toning the spinal nerves and promoting proper function of the digestive system. It also stretches out the part of the Liver Meridian that runs along the inner thighs, releasing blockages and enabling smooth energy flow.

NOTE: *For further stretching and relaxation, take several full breaths in each position before releasing it.*

1. Sit on the floor with your right leg stretched out to the side and your left leg bent and tucked in.

2. Place your right hand behind the arch of your right foot. Breathe in and stretch your left arm up, bending from the waist as you reach your hand over your head to your right foot. Hold for as long as comfortable while focusing on stretching your left side as much as possible. Exhale and return to your original position.

3. Switch your legs and repeat on the opposite side. Repeat at least twice for each side.

4. Now sit up with your spine straight and spread your legs apart.

5. Place your right hand on the left side of your rib cage. Breathe in and bend from the waist as you bring your left hand over to your right foot. Hold for as long as is comfortable while focusing on stretching your left side as far as you can. Exhale and return to your original position.

6. Repeat on the opposite side. Repeat at least twice for each side.

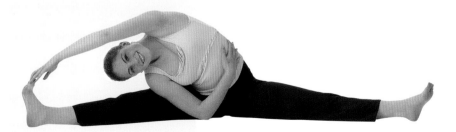

BUTTERFLY FORWARD BEND

BENEFITS: This exercise stretches the hip joints, inner thighs, and back. It also relieves tightness in the chest and promotes deep and full breathing.

NOTE: *Keep your back straight rather than curving it as you bend.*

1. Sit and put the soles of your feet together. Keep your back straight and your shoulders relaxed.

2. Hold your ankles as you gently bounce your upper body forward about 10 times.

3. Now inhale and bend your upper body forward. Try to touch your chest to your feet and your head to the floor.

4. Exhale and sit up. Expand your chest as you return to the starting posture.

5. Repeat several times.

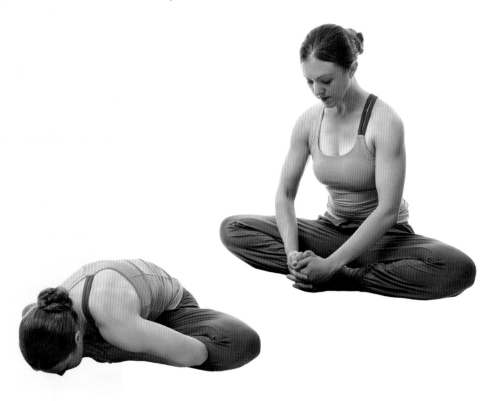

HIP BOUNCE

BENEFITS: Energy circulates in the hips and waist, and the organs are strengthened.

NOTE: *Relax your waist and lower extremities while performing this exercise.*

1. Lie on your back with your knees bent and your feet flat on the floor, parallel to each other and hip-width apart.

2. Place your palms down on the floor, slightly away from your sides.

3. Raise your hips and bounce them up and down, tapping your hips and lower back against the ground for about 3 minutes.

4. As you continue to practice this exercise, extend the time that you bounce your hips.

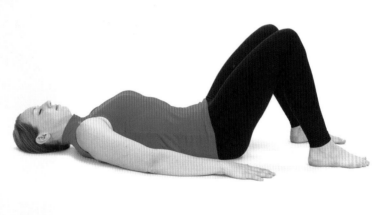

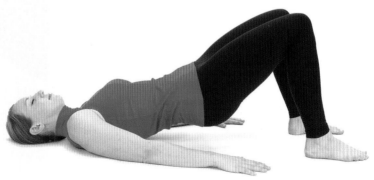

TOE TAPPING

BENEFITS: This exercise helps increase circulation to the lower extremities and balances water and fire energy in the body. It will also help you have deeper and more peaceful sleep. If you suffer from insomnia, try doing this exercise just before bedtime.

NOTE: *You can perform this exercise from either a lying down or a sitting position. If sitting, support yourself by placing your hands on the floor behind you and if lying down, rest them on your abdomen.*

1. Lie on your back or sit with your feet together.

2. Flex your ankles, keeping your heels together.

3. Tap your big toes together, then open your feet so that your little toes tap the floor. Repeat as rapidly as you can. Emphasize your exhalation.

4. Begin with 100 repetitions and increase that number as you practice more.

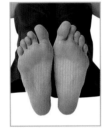
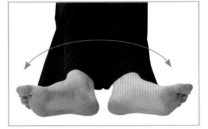

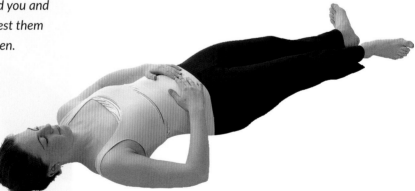

ROLLING BACK

BENEFITS: This exercise lengthens and strengthens the muscles of the spine. It enhances the nervous system and promotes optimal functioning of the vital organs.

NOTE: *Let your neck and head stay relaxed and rhythmically follow the motion rather than leading the motion. This is best done on a lightly cushioned surface.*

1. Sitting with your knees bent, clasp your arms around your knees. Round your spine to form a C shape. Slightly lower your head. Relax your neck and your shoulders.

2. Gently roll backward, with your back softly touching the floor, to stimulate your spine.

3. Slowly and gently return to the Step 1 position.

4. Repeat 10 times.

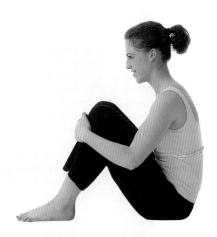

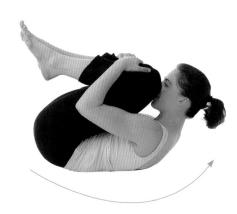

SHAKING HANDS AND LEGS

BENEFITS: This is helpful for energy circulation in the whole body as well as for relaxation, especially before bed or when feeling too tired.

NOTE: *Try to shake your entire arm and leg. You can shake vigorously or gently. The more tense your body or the busier your mind, the harder you should shake, within the limits of your physical condition.*

1. Lie on your back and raise your arms and legs straight up above you.

2. Shake your arms and legs for 3 minutes.

3. Let your arms and legs drop back down. Relax and exhale as you feel the subtle vibrations in your body.

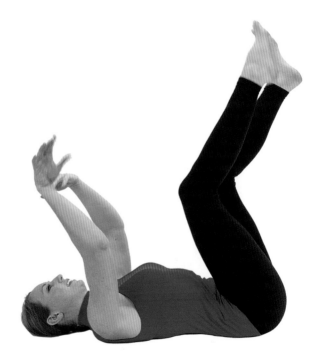

WRAP-UP EXERCISES
WHOLE BODY STRETCH

BENEFITS: This exercise strengthens the abdominal muscles, stretches the spine and back muscles, and promotes blood circulation. The swinging movement keeps the intestines in their proper place and relieves constipation.

NOTE: *Because of its energizing effect, this stretch is most often used as a finishing exercise. It's good to do it just after breathing posture sequences.*

1. Lie on your back and lock your fingers together. Breathe in and extend your arms above your head, fingers clasped. Point your toes downward and stretch your entire body. Exhale and relax. Repeat 3 times.

2. Flex your toes and bring your ankles together.

3. Slide your arms and legs to the left side and then to the right side. Synchronize your movements so that your upper and lower body move together.

4. Repeat several times.

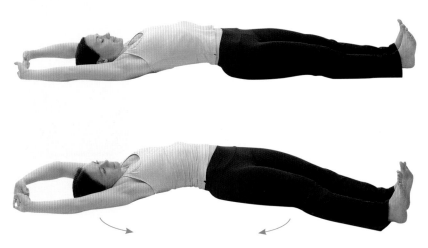

CROSSING LEGS TO FINGERS

BENEFITS: This exercise limbers the legs and hips, relieves tension in the back and torso, and increases spinal flexibility. It also tones abdominal muscles and massages a number of internal organs, including the liver and intestines.

NOTE: *Don't twist your lower back or pelvis farther than is comfortable. Stop if the pose causes any pain.*

1. Lie on your back with arms extended to the side at a 90-degree angle to your torso, with your palms facing upward.

2. Inhale. Lift your left leg to form a 90-degree angle with the ground.

3. Continuing to hold your breath, cross your left leg over your torso to touch your right fingers. Simultaneously turn your head to the left and gaze at your left hand.

4. Exhale. Return to the Step 1 position and perform the exercise on the opposite side.

5. Repeat twice.

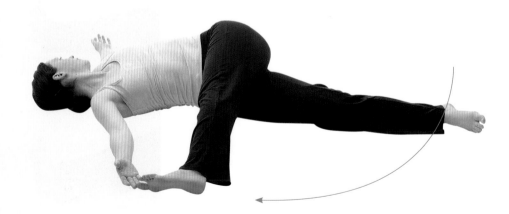

LIFTING LEGS OVER HEAD

BENEFITS: This exercise stretches the whole body and strengthens back, shoulder, and arm muscles while also releasing tension. It increases the flexibility of the spine in both the back and the neck and massages the internal organs by compressing the abdomen.

NOTE: *When you practice this stretch, make sure to keep your spine pushed up and your knees straight.*

1. Lie comfortably on your back. Rest your arms on the floor at your sides with your palms down.

2. Inhale. Keep your feet together as you slowly raise them off the floor, lifting your legs over your head until your toes touch the floor.

3. Hold this position for a few seconds. You can maintain this stance by supporting your lower back with your hands or by holding your feet with your hands.

4. Exhale and return to the Step 1 position. Repeat 3 more times.

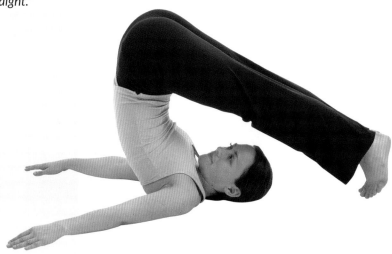

UPPER BODY LIFT

BENEFITS: This exercise strengthens the lower back and the lower torso with a powerful backward stretch as the abdominal organs are toned and massaged. This works well as a finishing exercise.

NOTE: *If you suffer from lower back pain, perform this exercise very carefully and gently.*

1. Lie on your stomach. Place your palms on the floor by each shoulder. Inhale and slowly raise your upper body, using your arms for support.

2. As you raise your upper body, lift your head up and hold it in this position while you concentrate on your spine.

3. Exhale and return to the Step 1 position. Repeat several times.

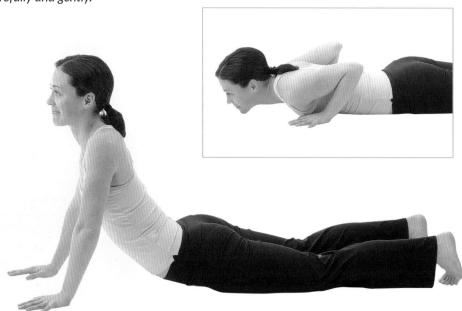

RELAXATION & MEDITATION

When energy fills up the lower dahnjon, our bodies and minds are naturally revived. After practicing Meridian Exercises, the circulation of energy and blood increases so that we can achieve a more deeply relaxed and meditative state.

Meditation involves focusing the mind and observing ourselves in the moment. It can take us deeper inside ourselves, beyond the illusions created by our thoughts and senses, so that we experience everything in its truest form. In short, meditation is a stilling of the mind. Practitioners of Body & Brain Yoga are encouraged to do this by focusing the mind on energy. The aim is to channel the mind's attention into a single focus, beginning with the feeling of energy between the hands. This sensation later grows to include energy flowing through and around the whole body. Through careful concentration, we can subdue the mind's endless stream of random thoughts and become fully present in the body.

If you find yourself distracted by a single stray thought, simply bring your mind back to the feeling of energy. Don't take any more note of it; simply refocus. Let distractions come and go without engaging them. Eventually your mind, breath, and energy will become one.

Once you are connected to your breath and energy, it becomes easy to return to your body. Most of the time, we experience life through the body without really being aware of that body. A web of busy inner dialogue runs through our mind, and we're so mesmerized by our ideas about the world that we miss out on much of the body's direct sensory experience. In Body & Brain Yoga, we use the body as a tool to reawaken ourselves to sensations. Becoming aware of physical sensations is a necessary prerequisite to mindfulness, because such sensations are linked to feelings and thoughts. They are the foundations of the process of consciousness.

Being mindful of the sensations in our bodies doesn't mean standing apart like distant witnesses. Rather, we directly experience what is happening in our bodies, and we feel the energy that flows through when we focus on them. Awakening to our bodies lets us experience the physical world fully, with all its anxieties, confusions, and pleasures, instead of living in a world of thoughts alone. Watching your body means asking yourself, "How does it actually feel to be anxious, angry, or happy? What is the texture of the experience?"

RELAXATION
BODY SCANNING

Relaxation of body and mind is the beginning of the path to a fully meditative state. The first step on this path is bringing our awareness into the body. Just by taking this step, body and mind start to relax and breathing deepens. Then sensations of energy can be felt more strongly and completely. Simply scanning all parts of the body with the mind shifts each part into a relaxed state.

When we are fully relaxed, we can move in any posture and remain relaxed in both body and mind. For most people, it's best to begin the relaxation process lying down so that no muscles are being used to support the body, allowing them to relax completely. Doing other exercises that release tension from the muscles—such as Meridian Exercises, breathing postures, cardiovascular exercises, or strength training—before using a relaxation technique enables the mind to feel the body more deeply and relax more quickly.

1. Lie on the ground with spine and neck as straight as possible. Close your eyes and look down into your body. Breathe comfortably.

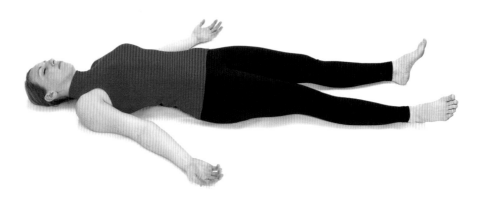

2. In your mind's eye, scan your entire body from head to toe. Begin with the crown of your head and move slowly down your body without missing any part. Include organs in your scan, such as your brain, heart, and stomach.

3. Notice how your body feels, without attaching to that feeling. If you encounter any tension, release it by exhaling through the mouth. You may feel your body becoming soft, and as if it is sinking down into the surface beneath it.

4. After scanning your entire body, return your awareness to your lower dahnjon. Leave it there for a couple of minutes to deepen your breathing and gather energy there.

FEELING ENERGY

JIGAM

Relaxed concentration is a prerequisite for feeling the flow of energy. We usually tense up when we concentrate, and when we stop concentrating, we let our thoughts wander without direction. Relaxed concentration may sound like an oxymoron. However, only when we can direct our consciousness while maintaining a relaxed state of body and mind can we feel the flow of energy.

To feel the energy, we need to turn the focus of our consciousness inward. We must separate ourselves from external distractions, thoughts, and emotions. We call this process Jigam, which literally means "stop emotion." The basic requirement for Jigam practice is determined concentration on the body, here and now.

We begin Jigam training with our hands because they are the most sensitive part of the body, letting us feel energy most easily. Once we are able to sense energy in our hands, it becomes easier to awaken this same sensitivity in other parts of the body, including the brain. The amount of time it takes to feel this energy for the first time varies from person to person, but with practice everyone will eventually succeed.

When we become used to feeling energy in our hands, we can maintain the sensitivity and the feeling without having to be in a specific position or environment. This means that it is possible to function in the everyday world in a clearer and calmer state of consciousness.

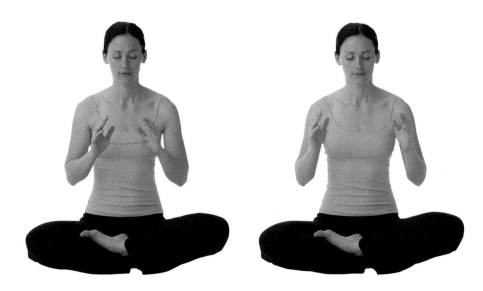

1. Sit in a half lotus position and straighten your back.

2. Place your hands on your knees with your palms facing up, then close your eyes. Relax your body, especially your neck and shoulders. Relax your mind. Inhale deeply and let go of any remaining tension while you exhale.

3. Raise your hands slowly to chest level, with your palms facing each other but not touching. Concentrate on any sensation you feel between your palms. You may feel warmth, tingling, or even your own pulse.

4. Now, part your hands by about 2 to 4 inches and concentrate on the space between them. Imagine that your shoulders, arms, wrists, and hands are floating in a vacuum, weightless.

5. Inhale as you pull your hands apart, then exhale and push them closer in again. Maintain your concentration as you feel the energy flow into and between your palms.

6. When the sensation becomes stronger, pull your hands farther apart and then push them closer together. Feel the sensation of energy expand and become stronger.

7. After a few minutes, return your hands to your knees, palms up. Breathe in and out 3 times, slowly and deeply.

8. Rub your hands together briskly and then gently sweep your hands over your face, head, neck, and chest.

FLOWING WITH ENERGY

DAHNMU

Dahnmu is a form of dancing with the natural flow of energy. This gentle dancing is an effective way to control and use energy. Practitioners usually experience energy as warmth, a tingling sensation, or a gentle vibration within the body. The energy usually begins in the hands through Jigam exercise and then gradually moves through the body until the entire body is responding in dance-like movements.

This exercise is particularly easy, since there's nothing to learn in the way of technique. The alignment of the body with energy is influenced by the participant's state of mind. The resulting Dahnmu might be expressed with motions that are fast or slow, restrained or passionate. It might include complex and intricate movements that you wouldn't normally make. When the rhythmic flow of energy is followed with movement, you dance naturally, ignoring long-repressed past inhibitions. These graceful motions come from deep within one's being as a perfect, spontaneous expression of vital energy. Out of these dance-like movements of self-expression, you begin to experience a gentle, dynamic meditation from a subconscious state.

As the dancing progresses, you can begin to feel joy and gratitude bubbling up from inside you. Tears may erupt, releasing emotions that had been locked in the chest. Experiencing Dahnmu brings forth a true understanding of freedom. Allowing spontaneous dance movements is the same as trusting the benevolent wisdom of energy. After realizing the way energy works, you can easily gain control of it and begin to use it at will.

1. Sit comfortably in a half lotus position. It is ideal to have background music that can naturally lead your body movement while you are practicing.

2. Repeat the Jigam exercise described earlier, gradually increasing the feeling of energy.

3. While immersing yourself in the feeling of energy through the motions of opening and closing your hands, you will feel your whole body move naturally. This is the beginning of Dahnmu.

4. Let the feeling of energy expand from your hands to your arms, shoulders, and torso. Allow your body to move naturally with the flow of the energy.

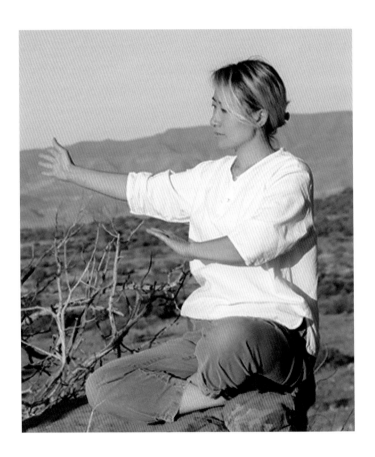

VISION MEDITATION

MINDSCREEN MEDITATION WITH LIFEPARTICLES

Our brains sometimes can't distinguish between reality and imagination. Imagine that you're taking a bite of a very sour lemon. Although you actually haven't eaten the lemon, you begin to salivate. As you can see from this example, our thoughts and emotions directly impact our bodies. That's why it is important to focus your mind intently on what you would like to bring into reality.

When you have discovered a desired goal, make up your mind that you will achieve it. Imagine that you have already made it happen, and believe that you will get to that point. Keep making detailed action plans and challenge yourself endlessly until you can see actual results.

During this process, imagination and belief in yourself play crucial roles. If you can vividly draw what you desire, then you'll be able to find plenty of ideas to make it come true. The imagination plays such a critical role because it's the foundation of creativity. Having desire is one thing; being able to imagine and implement that desire is another thing altogether. When we can clearly picture what we want, we can set goals and know which direction to take in order to reach them.

MindScreen Meditation is a type of vision meditation for drawing a desired state or goal on the inner screen of the mind as realistically as possible by using positive thoughts, emotions, and imagery. This picture becomes more powerful when energy is added to it. LifeParticles, the combination of energy, consciousness, and matter that is the most basic unit of all life, can be directed toward a goal by using the imagination. Sending LifeParticles to this

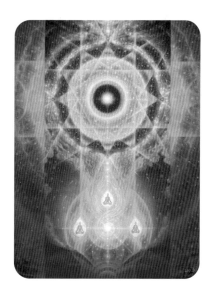

LIFEPARTICLE SUN

105

picture with the intention of creating something follows the principle of Shim Ki Hyul Jung—where the mind goes, energy gathers to create matter. LifeParticles are often visualized as golden or aquamarine particles of light coming from their source, which Ilchi Lee calls the LifeParticle Sun.

For this kind of visualization to be most effective, the entire energy system should be fully activated and the mind should be in a state of relaxed concentration. This meditation helps us apply the things we've gained from training to our daily lives.

1. Sit in a half lotus position and straighten your back. Sensitize yourself to energy by doing Jigam.

2. Once you feel the surrounding energy field, hold your hands on either side of your head without actually touching it. Feel the flow of energy emanating from your brain.

3. Spread your fingers apart and then bring them in again to expand the feeling of energy. Bring your hands closer to your head and push them farther out as you feel energy manifested as magnetic attraction and repulsion.

4. Let the movement of your hands, breath, and brain synchronize into a single rhythm. Imagine your body inflating and deflating with your breath. This form of energy meditation is known as Brain Jigam.

5. After a few minutes, rest your hands on your knees, palms up. Visualize the LifeParticle Sun, shown on page 105, in front of your forehead. See it coming into your brain and making your whole brain bright.

6. Then create a picture in your mind of what you want to be or achieve. Imagine in detail that it's already happened. Give yourself acknowledgment and a self-assuring message.

7. Visualize golden particles of light, LifeParticles, moving toward the picture you've created. See that image becoming more vivid.

8. Finally, sit calmly and focus on your breath for another minute more.

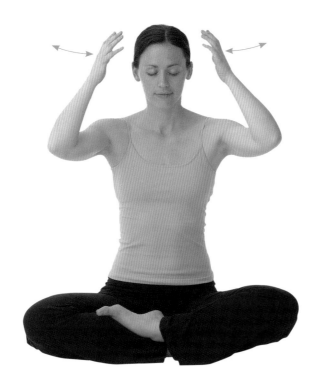

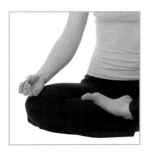
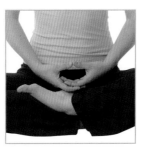

BRAIN WAVE VIBRATION

Sundo philosophy reveals that the body and brain can recover and maintain health when they follow their natural rhythms. We can remove disruptions to these rhythms by removing blocks to the flow of energy in our bodies and our brains. Brain Wave Vibration is the exercise that allows you to immerse yourself fully in the rhythm of life. Giving your body and mind over to your own internal rhythm is the key to this form of dynamic moving meditation.

Following your internal rhythm involves freeing your body and mind from how you usually move and think, how you think you should move and think, and how you believe others think you should move and think. In such a state of freedom, your energy flows freely and you can feel it more strongly. This free movement also sets your creativity free. You can see things in a new light.

Part of this new perspective comes from shaking free and releasing emotions and thoughts that had been hidden away in your body and brain, especially in your subconscious mind. As old thoughts and emotions come up, you become more aware of the patterns that may have been interfering with your conscious choices. This is the first step in changing those patterns.

Studies have shown evidence that Brain Wave Vibration helps you have less stress and more positive emotions[1]. They have also indicated that it lowers depression and improves vitality, mindfulness, and the ability to fall asleep faster[2]. It may also reduce levels of low-density lipo-protein cholesterol (LDL) and the expression of inflammatory genes, as well as help you feel less tired and lonely and more relaxed and focused[3]. Practitioners have attested that Brain Wave Vibration helps relax muscles and joints and slow down brain wave frequency. By helping to turn off chronic stress, Brain Wave Vibration lets your body's natural healing mechanisms work more effectively.

Moving meditation such as this will quiet your thoughts more quickly and easily than meditations for which you remain still. This exercise also helps you restore the optimal Water Up, Fire Down energy balance in your body.

Tapping & Shaking

1. This form of Brain Wave Vibration can be performed sitting or standing. In either case, make your back straight and pull in your chin slightly so that your spine and head are aligned. Relax your neck, chest, and shoulders.

2. Close your eyes and bring your focus to your lower abdomen. Make loose fists and use the pinky side to tap 2 inches below your navel, over your lower dahnjon. Alternate your fists for the tapping.

3. Once you find a comfortable rhythm, start shaking your head gently from side to side. Focus on the place where your skull and spine meet; use this point as a pivot. Let yourself relax from this point from your neck all the way down to your tailbone. Start slowly and gently. You can shake more rapidly as you relax and become comfortable; follow the feelings and needs of your body.

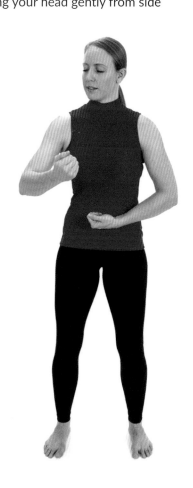

4. Imagine you are shaking out all of your thoughts. Exhale through your mouth, as if you were sending out any thoughts, tiredness, or hot energy.

5. Once your lower abdomen feels somewhat warmer, use your palms to pat any places on your body that seem blocked in order to open the energy points there.

6. After you feel fully relaxed, gradually slow your movements and then sit quietly. Calm your breathing while you bring your awareness back to your lower abdomen.

7. Try this exercise for 5 minutes to begin. Then gradually increase to 20 minutes or more.

Full-Body Vibration

1. Stand with your feet shoulder-width apart and your knees bent. Relax your shoulders, letting your arms hang forward a little.

2. Close your eyes, and begin to bounce your hips up and down in a comfortable rhythm. Expand this movement until your whole body is shaking up and down.

3. Exhale through your mouth as you bounce, releasing tension from your body. Continue until your body relaxes completely.

4. Now begin to make your own movements, following your natural rhythm. You can move strongly or gently—there's no right or wrong motion. Trust in the movements your body wants to make, without judgment or hesitation. Feel the sensations in your body.

5. Continue for 10 to 20 minutes, or until your body and mind feel calm yet full of vitality.

6. Gradually stop your motion, take a deep breath, and slowly sit down.

7. Bring your awareness to your lower dahnjon and breathe quietly for a few minutes.

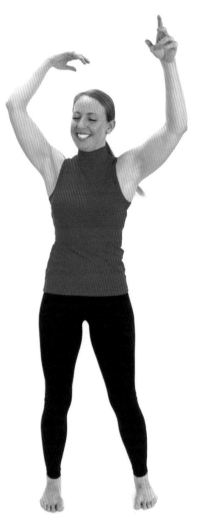

BOWING MEDITATION

Bowing is another form of moving meditation. While not used in regular Body & Brain Yoga classes, this meditation is an integral part of the practice. This single exercise enhances all three dahnjons and benefits body, mind, and spirit. The repetitive, full-body motion of Bowing Meditation loosens all the joints while opening all the meridian channels. Increased lower body and abdominal strength and better cardiovascular health are additional benefits. Like other forms of meditation, bowing helps calm and focus the mind, using the movement of the body and the energy within it as focal points.

Another point of focus for Bowing Meditation is the true self energy in the chest. Bowing while focusing there reinforces this energy, making it brighter and stronger. Each bow becomes a conversation with your true nature. As the movement lets you focus more deeply inside, you have the opportunity to see and accept everything about yourself, and you may experience feeling whole and complete.

Bowing Meditation is performed as a continuous motion, with one movement flowing into the next and one bow immediately following another. As you bow, let your breathing be natural; it will sync with the movements and grow deeper without conscious effort on your part. Experienced practitioners of Bowing Meditation may intentionally coordinate their breathing with their movements. They may also be able to feel the energy flow as they gather it with their hands and circulate it throughout their bodies.

1. Choose the number of bows you want to perform. Common numbers are 9, 21, 49, or 103.

2. Stand with your feet together and your palms together in front of the center of your chest.

3. Focus your mind on the lower dahnjon.

4. Move your hands downward and toward the sides of your body, straightening your arms.

5. Inhale as you turn your palms upward and move them up in a wide arc until you them together again over your head.

6. Keeping your palms together, slowly lower your hands in front of your chest.

7. Still keeping your palms together, bend forward at the waist about 90 degrees while keeping your legs straight.

8. Now raise your upper body slightly as you bend your knees and lower yourself into a kneeling position, with your toes on the ground and your ankles flexed. Sit with your weight on your heels. If it is difficult for you to do this safely, you can use your hands to steady yourself. Or lower one knee at a time to the ground while using your hands for balance.

9. Bend forward at the waist and place your palms on the floor so that you are on all fours. Straighten your ankles so the tops of your feet touch the ground.

10. Move your body down and back so that your buttocks touch your heels, your chest touches your knees, and your forehead and arms touch the floor. Go as far down as you can.

11. In this position, turn your palms upward and lift your hands, bending at the elbows as you exhale.

12. Now bring your palms back to the ground and raise yourself back up onto your hands and knees.

13. Flex your ankles and turn your toes under. Come up into a kneeling position as you bring your palms together in front of your chest.

14. Slowly lift yourself to a standing position to complete one bowing cycle. Use your hands for balance as you rise, if necessary. Continue this cycle until you complete the number of bows you've chosen.

Start Here

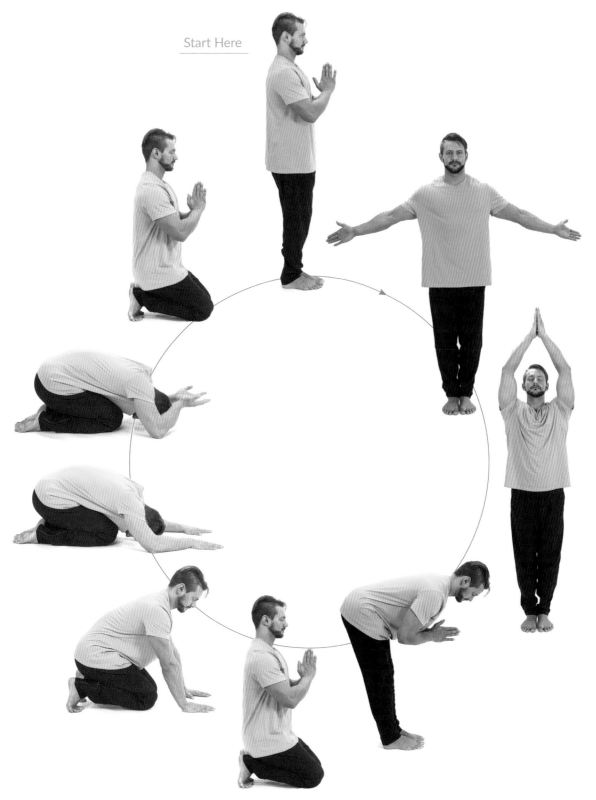

KIGONG & TAI CHI

Like Meridian Exercises, kigong (also spelled qigong, chigung, or chikyung) is an energy training method based on ancient Asian tradition that promotes the health of body and mind and harmonious living through conscious concentration, movement, and breathing. The principles underlying kigong form the basis of tai chi, which was originally developed as a martial art and involves set forms of movement.

Tai chi and kigong are both used to gather and circulate energy in the body and in the external environment. Feeling and circulating energy is like learning to swim. Water buoyancy is invisible and untouchable, but you can feel it and use it to float and swim freely. You feel and respond to the water, while at the same time, you are moving the water.

When you move naturally with the flow of energy, as in Dahnmu, and go deeper into that feeling, martial arts-like movements may naturally flow out of you. Tai chi is a natural extension of being deeply in tune with the energy of life. These movements can be strong or gentle, quick or slow. Using slow movements, however, enables you to concentrate on the energy more precisely and profoundly. It is from such movements that the various tai chi forms were developed. Most often, these are performed standing up.

By practicing tai chi, you develop the ability to move with the flow of energy throughout your daily life. This keeps the body in optimal health and vitality and the mind bright, positive, and peaceful. It makes it easier to distinguish thoughts, emotions, food, and other energies that can cause harm, letting you make healthier choices. Even more importantly, the fresh energy constantly coming through the body cleanses it of imbalances and toxic energy to bring it to a harmonious state. The purpose of kigong and tai chi in Body & Brain practice is not only to train the mind and body but also to become one with the flow of life and thereby benefit all life forms.

Dahngong

Dahngong is the most basic type of Body & Brain tai chi. As a martial art that is strong yet gentle, Dahngong has a compressed power within its softness. Even strong actions include movements in which you momentarily relax. Tremendous power is emitted in those instants, and energy is radiated.

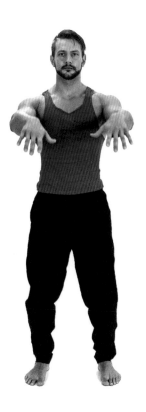

There are three main Dahngong forms—basic, accumulation, and circulation. Dahngong Basic Form is composed of the most frequently used and basic movements, hand techniques, leg stances, and energy circulation techniques. Strongly stretching arms and legs in this form corrects misaligned bones and muscles and creates fitness for the next level of practice. After mastering the basic form, you can move to the accumulation form, in which you learn how to make your upper body light while your lower body maintains its strength and firmness. When you've accumulated enough energy, you can advance to the circulation form.

One of the advantages of Dahngong is that rather than exhausting you, long periods of training can actually energize you. This is because energy keeps accumulating in the dahnjon during training as you move with the flow of energy. By adapting to the flow of energy to control and use it, you also can understand the mind—the essence of energy. In other words, Dahngong is a mental discipline for learning how to control yourself rather than being a tool for controlling or attacking an opponent.

You can only experience the true power of Dahngong when you practice it while feeling energy. If you aren't aware of the energy flow, then you are just making empty motions. After performing Dahngong with breathing, movement, and consciousness united in harmony, you may feel the body heat up, especially at the Jangshim and Yongchun points and the three internal dahnjons.

Controlling tension during Dahngong is important. Having excess muscle tension as you move doesn't allow energy to flow and doesn't let you move freely. On the other hand, ki is not generated if you are too relaxed and do the movements too gently. If you feel strength draining out of your body from doing Dahngong, you haven't yet found the right balance between tension and relaxation. This ideal balance consists of each Dahngong movement being generated by about 30 percent muscle strength and 70 percent energy power.

If you aren't relaxed enough, your lower dahnjon isn't strong, and/or you don't have Water Up, Fire Down energy circulation in your body, you may feel unstable or your breathing may be erratic during Dahngong. Doing other exercises first, such as Meridian Exercises, breathing postures, and Jigam, can prepare your mind and energy for the practice of Dahngong.

You can perform the Dahngong movements without needing to do them perfectly. Rather, practice moving with energy, with your body relaxed and comfortable. When you have more Dahngong practice, you can refine your motions and also widen and deepen your stance. Taking a wider stance and bending your knees more will help you develop greater flexibility, strength, and stability. Through practice, you also will be able to have a sense of stillness in motion in each and every movement.

DahnMuDo

DahnMuDo is an entire martial art form designed to enhance personal strength and integrity. The ultimate goal of DahnMuDo is to develop full mastership of body, mind, and spirit. This style of healing martial art includes kicks, hand strikes, held postures, strong forms, and soft forms. While some forms can be physically challenging, DahnMuDo is gentle enough to be practiced by anyone of any age. The forms are intentionally designed to avoid injury to the body, and the speed, strength, intensity, and height of the moves can be adjusted for each individual practitioner.

The main principle of movement in DahnMuDo is that the lower body remains strong and firm while the upper body is kept light and comfortable. All DahnMuDo movement is centered on the lower dahnjon and pivots around a pillar of energy through the center of the body. The hip joints must be relaxed, and the body's weight must be distributed evenly so that it rests solidly over the feet touching the ground. To develop lower body strength, practitioners work to hold a posture for extended periods of time. This also causes respiration to deepen and energy to collect in the dahnjon.

UNKIBOHYUNGGONG

One primary form in DahnMuDo used often in Body & Brain Yoga is a seven-posture form called Unkibohyunggong. This form adds hand movements to different leg postures (bohyung) to grow stability and strength in the lower body. The postures develop and stimulate the hemispheres of the brain as the left and right sides of the body move with balance and coordination. These postures also promote proper circulation of energy throughout the body. The training for each set is generally done for about one minute by beginners and about three to five minutes once practitioners are more comfortable with the postures. When moving from one set to the next, practitioners transition smoothly between postures, moving like water as they flow with universal energy. Since it trains the lower body so intensely, Unkibohyunggong also helps to build the lower dahnjon, the center of physical energy. This, in turn, leads to greater centeredness and clarity of mind.

Set One: Bow Stance (*Gungjeonbo*)
In Bow Stance, your front leg is curved like a bow and your back leg is straight like an arrow. The point is to feel contractive pressure on the pelvis and to align the angle of the hip joints correctly. This stance straightens the lower back, adjusts the spine and pelvis, and develops the strength of the back part of the thigh, spreading energy to the whole body.

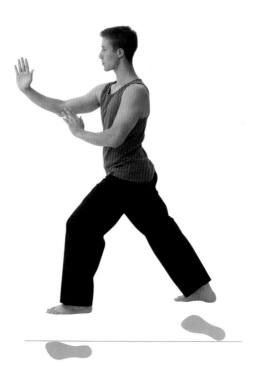

Set Two: Horse Stance (*Kimabo*)

For Horse Stance, stand with your feet parallel and about one and a half to two shoulder-widths apart. Bend your knees so that your entire weight rests firmly over the soles of your feet. This stance is effective for bringing energy down to the dahnjon as you concentrate your awareness there, taking advantage of the weight-bearing power of your feet.

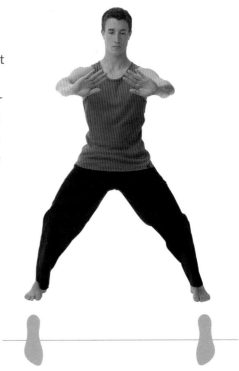

Set Three: Empty Stance (*Heobo*)

In this set, you rest all your weight on one foot while the other foot is "empty," with only the big toe touching the ground. The angle of the feet and legs toward each other puts a slight tension on the lower dahnjon. This allows energy to be accumulated quickly and the dahnjon to be rapidly strengthened. The contrast between the strength needed for the standing foot and the lightness needed for the empty foot helps develop quickness and resilience in the body.

45°

Set Four: Single Leg Stance (*Dongnibo*)
Like a crane standing elegantly on a single foot, the Single Leg Stance involves balancing on one leg with the knee of the other leg raised up to hip level. The raised foot rests beside the opposite knee with the ankle relaxed. This is effective for strengthening the legs and improving balance.

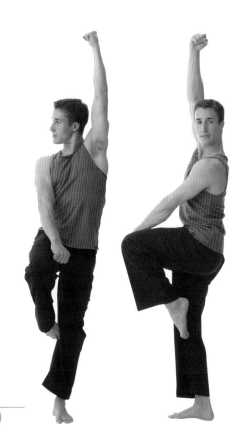

Set Five: Drop Stance (*Butwebo*)
For this stance, you extend one leg out to the side, stimulating the Gall Bladder Meridian at the side of your body. This fills one with confidence and trains the hip joint, while bending the other leg trains the thigh. Leg strength must be distributed evenly, since the legs take very different shapes in this stance. This is effective for causing energy to sink down into the lower body in a stable way to enable Water Up, Fire Down energy circulation.

Set Six: Sitting Stance (*Iljwabo*)

In martial arts, this stance is used to advance forward while keeping the body low. It looks as if you are taking a step, except your hips are sunk down, even until your front thigh is parallel to the ground. This enhances lower body strength and agility, because you can move in and out of the stance quickly.

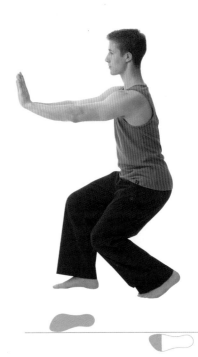

Set Seven: Cross Stance (*Jwabanbo*)

From Sitting Stance, turn your whole body in one direction as far as possible on the heel of one foot and the ball of the other foot and lower your stance until your knees are folding into each other, but not touching. This stance improves joint rotation, strengthens the muscles in the legs, and promotes active use of the lower back. It also develops strength, agility, and flexibility.

45°

Jikigong

Like other forms of tai chi and kigong, Jikigong is a dynamic meditation that matches movement with breathing and consciousness. Beginners can learn the movement first, then add the breathing for deeper awareness. In time, practitioners of this slow, flowing form may experience that there is stillness in motion and motion in silence.

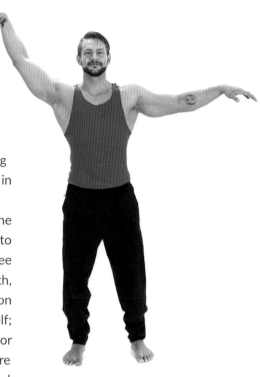

The Jikigong form is used to gather the energy of life from the earth and bring it into the body to activate and balance the three dahnjons. The lower dahnjon represents earth, or our physical existence; the middle dahnjon represents human, or our love and true self; and the upper dahnjon represents heaven, or our wisdom and insight. Therefore, there are three parts to this form: earth, human, and heaven. Each part shows you how to connect to and use the energy of the associated dahnjon. The heaven and earth parts accumulate energy in the body, while the human part circulates that energy.

Jikigong strengthens the lower body, deepens breathing, improves the sense of balance of the body, and revitalizes the sense of energy points such as the Myungmun, Jangshim, Yongchun, and Baekhwe. It helps develop a high level of mental concentration and achieve a detached, relaxed mind and a bold confidence.

The ultimate purpose of Jikigong is to bring about a great love for humanity and the earth. It's also meant to foster harmony among the different aspects of ourselves, between ourselves and others, and between ourselves and the earth.

Ilchi Kigong

Named after Ilchi Lee, the founder of Body & Brain Yoga, Ilchi Kigong consists of eight sets of movements for cultivating harmony among mind, body, heart, and nature. The movements are smoother and more flowing than some other kigong forms. Each set contains a philosophy for harmony of mind and body. It is important to understand the meaning of each set and to embody that meaning.

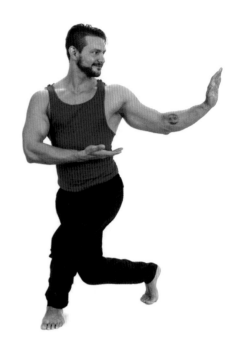

The philosophy and principles of Ilchi Kigong flow from creation to education to civilization. The principle of creation involves the concept that there are three intrinsic elements of harmony rather than a dichotomous structure of competition and confrontation. This is a universal principle of life and enlightenment in which humanity, nature, and the cosmos blend together. The principle of education involves sharing with the world and educating others in the philosophy of enlightenment. And according to the principle of civilization, this philosophy of enlightenment forms the basis of a social system in which all members live to perfect their lives as human beings.

Each of the eight sets involves turning, pushing, pulling, raising, and lowering each part of the body. Major movements include rotational motions and simple actions that angle the joints and squeeze out energy. Together, they produce a well-balanced physique.

There are many ways to practice Ilchi Kigong. You can learn the motions and then move very slowly while feeling energy. Or you can speed up the movements. Once you are familiar with the entire form, you can perform it from beginning to end or keep repeating one part to fully experience its energy. It is also a good idea to hold one of the positions for an extended period of time. The most common method of practice is to match breathing, movement, and awareness in order to feel stillness in the movement and flow as naturally as water.

The advanced practitioner is able to enter a blissful state of deep concentration through these simple motions. From such a state, you discover that infinite changes are possible from just one movement. Although the basic movements are simple, when you feel the spirit and energy in them, you will gain the confidence and power to change whatever you want in your life. This is the essence and true beauty of Ilchi Kigong.

Chunbushingong

Chunbushingong is a form that expresses through the body the meaning of the *Chun Bu Kyung*, a sacred text of ancient Korea. In just 81 characters, the *Chun Bu Kyung* speaks of the essential principles of the universe. It is the philosophical basis of the Korean Sundo tradition that is the root of Body & Brain Yoga.

Because 46 of the 81 characters of the *Chun Bu Kyung* are unique, so Chunbushingong has 46 different postures. Through each posture, the essence of that character can be felt. The postures are made one by one and combined with conscious breathing. They can be held for a few minutes each, or they can flow right into one another.

If you keep practicing, the energy of the *Chun Bu Kyung* will infuse your body and mind, making your body healthy and strong and your mind peaceful and harmonious. As your practice deepens, all the joints and energy points of your body will open to circulate energy completely. Furthermore, as the movements freely distribute the energy of the body and the energy of the universe, you will be able to experience a state of oneness with the universe.

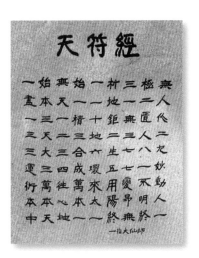

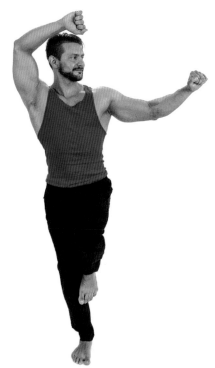

THE CHUN BU KYUNG

BREATHING

Breathing is an automatic process vital to survival. Yet it's also one of the most powerful bodily processes that can be consciously regulated. Through breathing, other automatic vital processes—such as heart rate and body temperature—can be intentionally influenced.

Breathing energizes the body through the taking in of oxygen and energy and through the facilitation of deep, revitalizing relaxation. This is especially important for the brain, which uses 25 percent of the oxygen the body takes in. If the brain doesn't receive adequate oxygen for even a few minutes, the brain suffers damage.

Not all breathing is equal, however. The breathing that is most beneficial is slow, deep, light, long, and natural, and it results in energy accumulation in the lower dahnjon. In order for breathing to be deep and long, the abdomen must be engaged in each breath. Babies naturally do this; as they breathe, their bellies rise and fall. As we get older, though, our breathing becomes shallower as the result of poor posture, stress, and tension. Instead of the abdomen being engaged with each breath, the chest rises and falls. In worse cases, even the chest is too stiff, and breathing comes from the throat.

Relaxation, then, is paramount for healthy breathing. It allows the abdomen to be engaged so that the diaphragm can move more easily to bring more oxygen into the body. It also lets energy flow and the mind focus inside the body, especially in the dahnjon, so that energy gathers there to create the ideal Water Up, Fire Down energy circulation. The more deeply relaxed and focused we are, the more stable and the longer our breathing becomes. Just by the mind focusing on the body and the breath, breathing begins to slow and deepen. This relaxes the body and slows brain waves, which further deepens and slows breathing in a natural feedback loop.

To gather energy in the lower dahnjon, through breathing or otherwise, the body needs to be properly positioned so that the energy coming in won't leak out. The hip joint, in conjunction with the tailbone, works as the valve for energy flow in the human body. Curling up the tailbone closes this valve because it helps form a proper angle for gathering energy while creating light tension in the dahnjon. Once the appropriate body position is taken, energy generated by breathing is naturally gathered at the dahnjon. This creates natural pressure around the abdomen, allowing proper energy circulation throughout the body to happen naturally.

Just as the energy system is supported by the proper positioning of tailbone and hips, so are the internal organs. The tailbone supports these organs because it is connected to many of the muscles that support the abdomen. The muscles of the lower abdominal cavity essentially form a "hammock" that supports all the surrounding organs, attaching in front to the forward pelvis and in back to the lower spine and tailbone.

Because of the importance of position, relaxation, and focus for healthy breathing and for stimulating the body's meridian system and effectively accumulating energy in the dahnjon, Body & Brain Yoga breathing techniques involve releasing tension from the chest and abdomen and breathing while in specific postures. The focus is on exhalation and proper positioning, and letting inhalation happen naturally without conscious or intentional control. With practice, the breathing postures change the body and brain so that we can breathe deeply and slowly even off the mat.

Deep, healthy breathing activates the body's rest and digestion functions to support its self-healing mechanisms. In addition to helping regulate physiological processes such as blood pressure and body temperature, deep breathing helps manage thoughts and emotions, even to the point of producing feelings of joy and well-being. Research has shown that conscious, deep breathing stimulates areas of the brain that are often dormant, and in experienced practitioners, it expands areas of the brain related to attention and sensory input processing. By transforming our breathing, we can make lasting changes to both body and brain.

Points to Remember for Breathing Practice

- For deep and natural breathing, any stress-caused blockage around the chest has to be opened. To open blockages, relax the chest and shoulders and focus on exhaling. To begin, exhale with your mouth open slightly. You can even make an "ah" sound in the throat to deeply release stagnant energy from inside the chest. Once your chest no longer feels stuffy or tense, it's better to breathe with your mouth closed and your tongue placed against the roof of the mouth. This closes the energy circuit formed by the Conception Vessel and Governing Vessel meridians and allows energy to accumulate and travel down into the lower dahnjon.

- Before, during, and after breathing training, feel your breath. Check whether your breathing is comfortable or uncomfortable, fast or slow, and whether it is moving your chest or abdomen. As you do that, you are communing with your body through breathing. Your awareness of body and mind increases as you feel your breathing, which will naturally become slower, deeper, and more comfortable.

- As your breathing deepens, you will begin to feel a pause between your inhale and exhale. This happens naturally; it's not an intentional pause. Even though your breathing has stopped for that moment, there is still energetic internal breathing taking place. This isn't actually stopping your breathing, but a momentary lingering of physical breathing. The longer this lingering moment becomes, the bigger a sense of peace grows. Distracting thoughts and emotions disappear, and your consciousness enters into a pure and clear state.

- As various phenomena take place, calmly watch the energetic sensations occurring in the body without attachment; keep your mind in your dahnjon. Whether you feel discomfort or a sense of bliss, or even if you see light or images, don't get caught up in these energy experiences. Instead, keep watching and remain steadily centered in your dahnjon. This is a form of Geumchok, or detaching from stimulation.

Chest Breathing

Body & Brain Yoga breathing techniques begin with Chest Breathing, which involves comfortable breathing as the chest rises and falls and the mind is focused on the chest area. Chest Breathing allows the chest to relax when it is too tight for abdominal breathing to be comfortable, or even possible.

Chest Breathing is often done in the following sequence of postures. Breathe in each posture for about two to three minutes.

For each posture, close your eyes and follow the concentration technique for Chest Breathing 1 until your chest is more relaxed. Then follow the technique for Chest Breathing 2. You don't have to do both Chest Breathing 1 and Chest Breathing 2 each time you practice Chest Breathing. Use Chest Breathing 1 for each session until Chest Breathing becomes more comfortable, then use Chest Breathing 2. But if you don't practice breathing for some time and your chest becomes tight again, you can go back to Chest Breathing 1 to release the stagnant energy.

CHEST BREATHING 1

With each inhale, imagine fresh energy coming into your body through the Dahnjoong point in the center of the sternum, and stagnant energy in the chest leaving the body through your fingertips with each exhale. Numbness, prickliness, coldness, and other such sensations all mean stagnant energy is being released. When you feel warmth in your chest and hands, it means the stagnant energy in the chest has been purified.

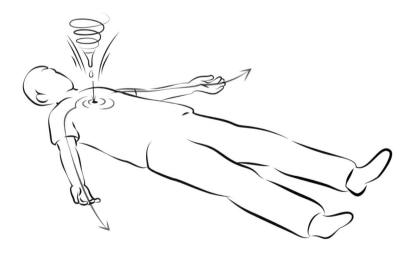

CHEST BREATHING 2

Imagine or feel the energy coming in through the Dahnjoong point with each breath then traveling down to the lower dahnjon each time you exhale. You may feel energy going past your hip joints and connecting down to the feet. You are fully engaged in Chest Breathing when you feel energy from your chest going down to the dahnjon and the dahnjon becoming warm.

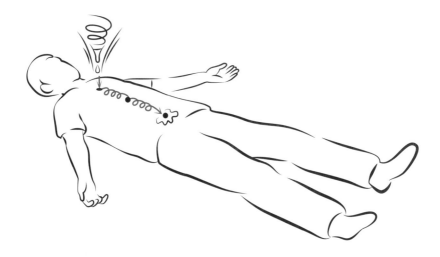

CHEST BREATHING POSTURE 1

1. Lie comfortably, face up, on a hard, warm surface. Spread your feet about shoulder-width apart, and move your arms out about 45 degrees from your sides, with elbows straight and palms up.

2. Curl your sacrum and hips in a little, just enough to feel a slight tension in your hips and abdomen.

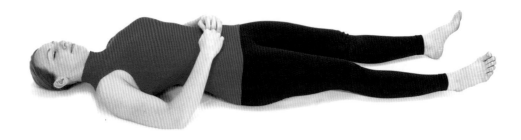

3. Tuck in your chin slightly so that your neck and spine stretch and relax. This will let energy flow down easily and bring focus to the dahnjon. Use a pillow under your head if your chin tends to lift up.

CHEST BREATHING POSTURE 2

1. From Posture 1, bring your hands to your lower abdomen. Form a triangle with your fingers, with your thumbs meeting at the navel.
2. Raise your knees but keep your feet on the ground, hip-width apart.
3. Keep your sacrum and hips tucked in and your chin slightly down.
4. Do Intestinal Exercises in synchronization with each breath.

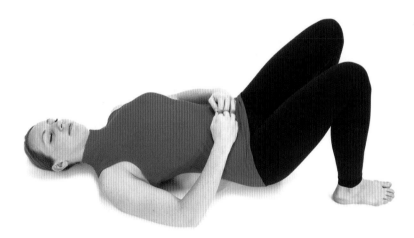

CHEST BREATHING POSTURE 3

1. From Posture 2, raise the hips until you make a straight line between your knees and shoulders, or as close to this as possible, depending on your flexibility and strength.
2. Continue to do Intestinal Exercises in synchronization with each breath.

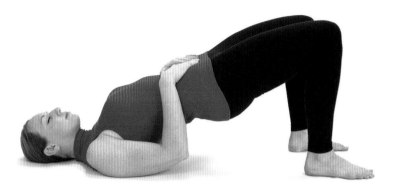

CHEST BREATHING POSTURE 4

1. From Posture 3, lower your hips and raise your feet to make right angles at the hips, knees, and ankles.

2. Tuck in your hips and tailbone, lengthening the lower back; have your tailbone touch the floor if that is comfortable. Keep your shoulders relaxed and your chin tucked in.

3. Adjust the angle of your lower legs so that you do not feel tension in your legs. You should feel more weight on your abdomen than your legs. The Yongchun will open and you will feel energy enter through your feet. Sense the pressure and energy gathering to the dahnjon.

4. Continue to do Intestinal Exercises in synchronization with each breath.

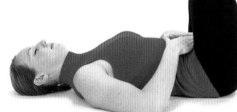

CHEST BREATHING POSTURE 5
Return to Posture 1

Dahnjon Breathing

The most important part of Dahnjon Breathing is creating a sensation of strong, warm energy in the lower dahnjon. At first, you may not feel any sensation there. This may be due to energy channels being blocked or your sense of energy not being fully developed. With practice, however, the warmth of the energy moving inside the abdomen will become apparent. When you have a feeling of heat in the abdomen, the location of that heat is the dahnjon. Concentrate on that point. As your awareness of the dahnjon increases, you will feel more energy and heat, and the feeling of heat may change into a magnetic or electric sensation.

When the dahnjon feels warm, imagine an energy ball in there. Deepen your breathing and the energy ball will become larger and denser. Soon the abdominal area will be filled with that ball of energy. Through the following postures and techniques, your breathing can become natural, deep dahnjon breathing.

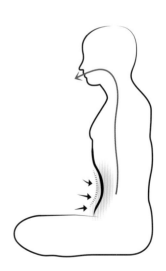

Hold each posture for three to five minutes, until your body relaxes and your breath deepens. If holding the posture is painful or too difficult, change to the next posture. Do not use overly strenuous postures. You can also use one of the meditation postures shown.

DAHNJON BREATHING 1

Perform each posture while focusing on the abdominal muscles. Feel them push out as you inhale and pull in as you exhale. While you are breathing, only move the lower abdomen. If the upper abdomen moves first, it's because the abdomen is too tense. Doing Intestinal Exercises fully focused on the lower abdominal muscles should help alleviate this (see page 65).

Breathe in a steady rhythm at a comfortable rate, making your lower abdomen swell up like a balloon. After doing Dahnjon Breathing for some time, you may feel warmth and a sense of space in the muscles surrounding the lower abdominal area. Then a sense of pressure will gather in the center of your dahnjon. Imagine an energy ball there— that is your energy center.

DAHNJON BREATHING 2

Perform each posture while focusing deep into the lower abdomen, on the dahnjon, rather than focusing on the movements of the abdominal muscles as in Dahnjon Breathing 1. Feel any changes in the energy center as you expand and contract from the dahnjon. Feel energy being accumulated in the dahnjon. The warmth and a sense of fullness in your dahnjon will become stronger and may spread around your waist.

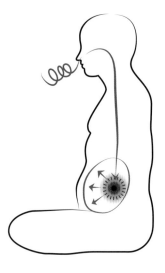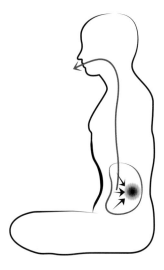

DAHNJON BREATHING POSTURE 1

RELAXATION

1. Lie on your back on a hard, warm surface.

2. Squeeze your legs tightly together, then completely relax them. They will part naturally. Your feet should be about 30 to 45 degrees from the floor.

3. Place your middle fingers very lightly on your Kihae energy point 2 inches below your navel. Do not press down, since the dahnjon is sensitive to the slightest sensation. Keep your elbows resting comfortably on the floor. If they lift up off the floor, let your hands slide down the sides of your abdomen until your elbows are on the floor.

4. Close your eyes and completely relax your body, especially the upper body, chest, and shoulders.

5. Gently curl your tailbone up, letting your lower back touch the floor as much as possible. As your tailbone curls, imagine creating a bowl in which your dahnjon can collect energy; try not to tense your legs as you do so. You will automatically feel slight tension in your lower abdomen. Find a body angle that helps you breathe the most naturally and comfortably.

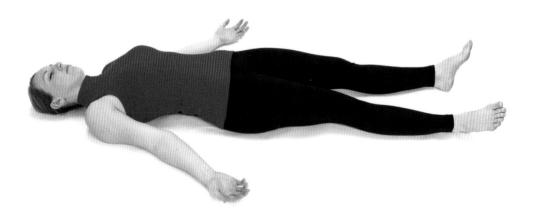

ACCUMULATION

1. Curl your tailbone upward, creating mild tension around the lower abdomen. Raise both legs with hips and ankles bent at a 90-degree angle and your knees bent at about 110 degrees so that they are slightly higher than your knees. To curl your tailbone in this posture, start by bringing your knees closer to your chest. Feel the tailbone lifting and the back touching the floor before readjusting the hips to a 90-degree angle.

2. Make your knees about a fist-width apart and your ankles slightly wider. Don't make the distance between the knees greater than the distance between the ankles, or energy will leak out.

3. Make your feet parallel. This helps keep the hip joints in the correct position for energy accumulation.

4. Flex your ankles by pushing your heels out. Don't curl the toes, as this creates blockages in the ankles.

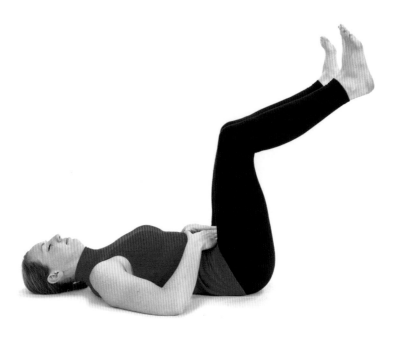

5. To accumulate more energy, you can also raise your arms so that your hands are above your shoulders, with your elbows slightly bent. Flex your wrists to stimulate the Jangshim points, and point both palms toward the ceiling. This posture is also known as Sleeping Tiger.

6. At first you may find that even holding the posture is difficult. With time and practice, however, you will breathe deeply and comfortably while holding the proper posture. You may feel a stream of energy flowing out from Yongchun point on the soles of your feet. This means that energy channels and points in your soles have been activated.

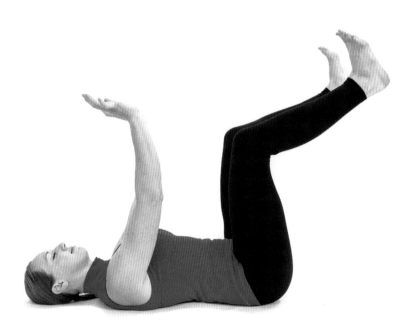

CIRCULATION 1

1. Lie down and slowly stretch and straighten both legs up in the air to the best of your ability. Firmly hold onto the heels, front, or sides of your feet. Straighten your knees as much as possible. If you can't do that, try to hold on to your ankles, calves, or the backs of the knees to keep from raising your shoulders or causing tension there.

2. Completely relax your chest and shoulders. Keep your head on the floor, your chin tucked in slightly, and your lower back as close to the floor as possible.

3. Flex your ankles and push out your heels to fully stretch the Bladder and Kidney Meridians on the back side of your body. You're likely to sense vibration as these meridians open.

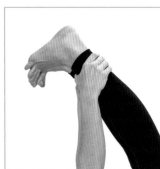

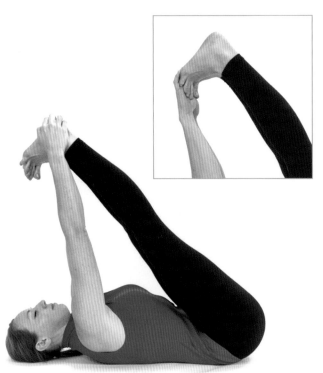

DAHNJON BREATHING POSTURE 4

CIRCULATION 2

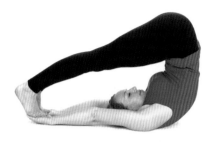

1. Starting from the previous posture, bring both legs completely up over your head.

2. Keep your heels pushed out as you stretch and straighten your knees. Feel the stretch along your spine, even if this means you can't keep your knees straight. If you are unable to straighten your knees, just flex your ankles back. It's okay if your toes can't touch the floor.

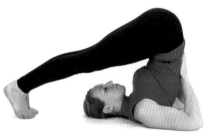

3. Your arms should remain stretched out above your head, holding your feet, in order to promote proper energy circulation.

4. Relax your shoulders as much as you can. If you feel some pressure in your chest, exhale more strongly.

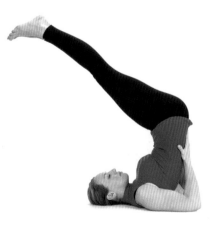

5. Connect the weight of the legs to the dahnjon as a sense of pressure. If your breathing doesn't come down to the dahnjon, don't bring your legs all the way back. Feel the Yongchun and Jangshim opening and your energy system opening.

Note: This posture should be avoided by anyone who is in weak physical condition, pregnant, or obese, or who has a spinal disk injury. In these instances, use Dahnjon Breathing Posture 2 or 3 instead.

RELAXATION AND ACCUMULATION

1. Bring your feet down to the floor with knees bent. For stronger energy accumulation, rest your legs on the floor in either a cross-legged or a half lotus position, or by putting your feet together as shown. You can also keep your legs straight instead.

2. Place your hands on your dahnjon in the shape of a triangle, with thumbs meeting at the navel and index fingers touching.

3. Curl your tailbone, pushing your lower back gently to the floor.

4. Release tension from the shoulders and chest. You will feel your lower back become more relaxed and comfortable and your legs become very light.

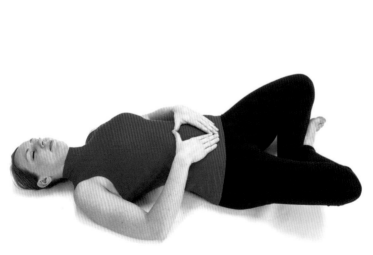
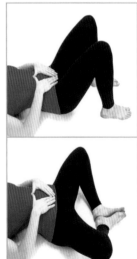

BREATHING

Myungmun Breathing

As Dahnjon Breathing deepens, it naturally develops into Myungmun Breathing. This involves the same postures as Dahnjon Breathing. The difference is that in Myungmun Breathing, the Myungmun energy point, which is found in the spine behind the navel, acts as the nose and the dahnjon acts as the lungs. This further enhances lower dahnjon energy development and Water Up, Fire Down energy circulation. Visualization and a strong sense for the energy in the body are important for Myungmun Breathing.

As you inhale during Myungmun Breathing, you imagine fresh energy gently and slowly entering the Myungmun, or you feel it with your energy sense. The energy reels in at a 45-degree angle and goes into the dahnjon, where it circulates in a spiral from the back of the body to the front, like the shell of a snail. At the same time, the abdomen gently expands out and down at a 45-degree angle. As energy comes in, you can eventually feel a marble of energy forming in the center of the dahnjon. On exhaling, stagnant energy leaves the body through the Myungmun, creating a stream of energy flowing along the channel between the dahnjon and the Myungmun.

During this exercise, your breaths will become longer. Your large and small intestines may automatically start moving as they soften and purify. Very pure energy is produced, and you become immersed in deep meditation.

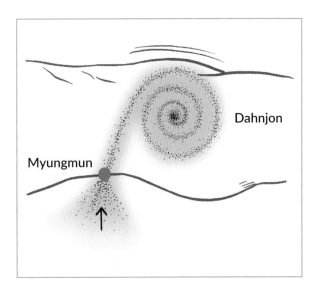

Sitting Breathing Posture

While the breathing posture sequences presented in this book are powerful, as your breathing practice deepens, you can simply choose one posture that works best for you at any given time. Using this posture, you can move from Chest Breathing to Dahnjon Breathing to Myungmun Breathing, or just do the type of breathing you need for your condition at the moment. One standard posture in any meditation practice that you can use is the simple half lotus posture shown below.

HALF LOTUS POSTURE

1. Sit with knees bent and one leg resting on top of the other.

2. Straighten your spine, with hips tilted back slightly and your chin tucked in slightly. Relax your shoulders and arms.

3. Place your hands on your knees, palms up. Or you can bring the tip of the thumb, index, and middle fingers together or put both hands on the dahnjon to form a triangle around the Kihae. Relax your chest muscles.

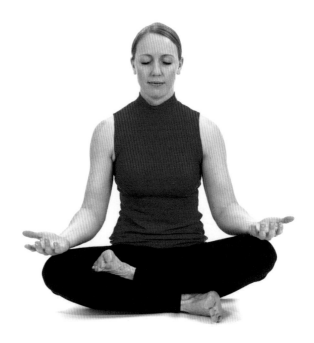

ENERGY POINT HEALING

All Body & Brain Yoga exercises stimulate and open meridian channels and energy points, but some activate them more directly through pressing and rubbing. By targeting specific points, you can concentrate on areas that are particularly powerful or need special attention. At the same time, this specific stimulation sends signals to the brain, informing it of areas of imbalance. Then the natural healing processes of the brain and body can work more effectively to address physical, emotional, mental, and spiritual issues related to those points.

BHP Energy Healing

In Body & Brain Yoga, the technique for finding and stimulating energy points is called BHP Energy Healing. This technique focuses on points on the head and just under the cuticles of the fingernails and toenails, because these are the most immediately and powerfully effective. These points correspond to all the other parts of the body, as well as our emotional, energetic, and spiritual condition. In BHP Energy Healing, you search for painful or tender points, because pain indicates blocked energy there and in related areas, which also correspond to emotional and mental issues that need to be solved. The more painful a point, the more that healing is needed. These Brain Education Healing Points (BHPs) offer an opportunity to restore internal balance and a connection between body and brain.

1. Find BHPs by pressing with a clean fingernail or a slightly pointed (but not sharp) tool. Start by pressing points on your head and then press below the cuticles on all your fingernails and toenails. Avoid any area with a cut, bruise, or open sore.

2. When you encounter a tender point, gently and repeatedly press and release on that spot for about a minute, or until the pain stops. Adjust the pressure as needed—it shouldn't hurt too much.

3. As you press, be aware of the sensations in your body, starting with the feeling of pressing that point. When you are very aware of your body and your energy, you may feel the tension releasing around that point; you may feel a release of tension and energy in other parts of your body as well. You may also experience emotional changes or particular thoughts and memories.

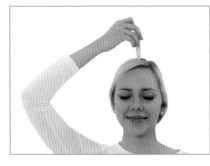 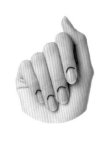 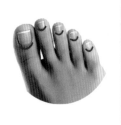

You may even feel Water Up, Fire Down occurring in your body, or a clear and light feeling in your brain. Rather than resisting the pain or any changes you experience, accept everything you sense, just as it is.

4. Exhale through your mouth as you press in order to release stagnant energy. This will also help with the pain.

5. Move from point to point until you have finished checking your head, fingers, and toes. You may have many BHPs or just a few. The number varies with the individual as well as one's condition at any given time.

6. Rest and breathe for a few moments afterward. Keep your focus inward, and note the changes in your physical, mental, and emotional states.

7. Whenever you have time, go back to the spots where you felt the most intense pain—about 3 to 5 times a day.

Belly Button Healing

Belly Button Healing focuses on one powerful acupressure point—the belly button. In Asian medicine, this point was traditionally used to revive people who fainted. It is also a reflexology point through which other parts of the body can be healed. The belly button lies near the lower dahnjon, so stimulating it also stimulates and accumulates energy in this important energy center.

Although on the outside the navel is only a scar left by the umbilical cord after birth, its location has importance for healing the body and brain. Beneath it in the abdomen are major blood vessels, lymph nodes, the digestive tract, and the reproductive organs. Thirty percent of the body's blood flows through the abdomen at any given moment. Major hormones such as serotonin and dopamine, which affect mood, reward, and digestion, are also produced there. A network of connective tissue links the belly button to the entire torso.

Pressing the belly button repeatedly relaxes the organs and connective tissue in the abdomen, allowing blood and lymph to flow better and the diaphragm to move deeper into the abdomen so that more oxygen enters with each breath. This also releases pain in the joints and back. The pressing pushes blood and lymph through their vessels and food and waste through the intestines. This rhythmic motion, like that in Brain Wave Vibration, slows down brain waves and activates the body's rest and digest functions via the parasympathetic nervous system.

1. You can do Belly Button Healing while standing, sitting, or lying down. Cover your navel with clothing or a towel.

2. Gently rub your palm clockwise on your abdomen for a minute to relax your body and mind.

3. Use your fingers or a blunt tool to repeatedly and gently press the belly button through the cloth covering. To use your fingers, bring together the index, middle, and ring fingers of both hands.

4. Bring your attention inside yourself and feel the sensations in your lower abdomen. Observe the changes in your body.

5. Let your mouth open slightly, and continuously breathe out the stagnant energy in your body.

6. Continue pressing for about 3 to 5 minutes or longer.

7. Afterward, spend some time breathing comfortably as you observe how your body feels. Notice how your breath becomes deeper.

Note: A special tool was developed by Ilchi Lee for practicing Belly Button Healing most effectively. The ergonomic and natural design of the Belly Button Healing Wand allows practitioners to relax their shoulders and use less strength for pressing the navel. This tool can also be used to massage other parts of the body.

WORKSHOPS & RETREATS

In addition to daily classes, Body & Brain Yoga offers workshops that can help you propel your practice forward and reach your highest potential. When combined with regular class attendance, these workshops let you experience deeper relaxation and a greater sense of energy and overall well-being. Most people find that even regular classes take on greater meaning and effectiveness after they've participated in a workshop.

ESSENTIAL WORKSHOPS

Initial Awakening

In order to develop a stronger connection between your body and your brain, this basic workshop shows you how to observe your body, thoughts, and emotions while learning to sense and strengthen your lower dahnjon. It will help you open up energy pathways and awaken your energy sense. You will be able to experience your body's energy system directly and feel how it works.

Finding True Self

The Finding True Self workshop focuses on the middle dahnjon to help you connect with the core of who you truly are and discover your inner power. It helps you let go of any anger and grief you may be holding and take a look at your thoughts, patterns, and habits. Through the workshop activities, you will generate enough energy and focus to be able to feel the answers to the important existential questions of "Who am I?" and "What do I want?" The workshop's physical exercises, group interactions, meditations, and self-reflections will help you open a path toward greater and deeper understanding of yourself, your motivations, and your potential.

International Brain Education Leadership Workshop

An International Brain Education Leader (IBEL) is someone who uses Brain Education to discover their greatest selves and solve their own problems as the leaders of their lives. This workshop takes you through essential Brain Education training. In the process, you gain the ability to read your current condition and learn how to apply Brain Education to your life. IBELs embody Brain Education principles, contributing to a happier, healthier, and more harmonious world.

IN-DEPTH COURSES

Brain Management Training

Managing your brain is the key to managing your life. Brain Management Training teaches you how to power up your brain and your energy system with simple yet powerful Brain Education techniques. You learn how to manage your brain for better health, more energy, and greater insight and self-discipline. The way you process information and experience your life is changed for the better. In order to fully absorb the techniques and become a positive influence in their families and communities, participants also engage in teaching.

Energy Healing Course

The Energy Healing Course provides in-depth experience in using Body & Brain Yoga's energy healing tools. You learn how to apply these tools to improve your own health and use them on others to help them activate their natural healing power. You develop your energy awareness, sensitivity, and strength. In addition to mind-body exercises, you learn how to use simple devices common to Body & Brain Yoga centers, such as the LifeParticle Card, Belly Button Healing Wand, HSP Wooden Pillow, and Bird of the Soul Essential Oil.

Dahn Master Course

This intensive workshop is for people who want to be Body & Brain Yoga instructors and dedicate themselves to self-mastery and their chosen purpose. Program benefits include developing a clearer goal and a sustained focus on that goal; increased capacity for acceptance, understanding, and compassion; and enhanced powers of discipline and self-management.

DahnMuDo Martial Art

The DahnMuDo Martial Art workshop takes you through a full curriculum of this non-combative, healing martial art. It involves several multi-day sessions and a progression through martial art belts all the way to a black belt. Through the practice of DahnMuDo, you can master spreading accumulated energy throughout your body. You also learn how to use your body to enhance your mental strength while gaining a sense of personal integrity.

Meditation Retreats

Body & Brain Yoga leads meditation tours designed to facilitate deeper self-exploration through an intimate connection to nature. You can visit such beautiful natural settings as the red rocks of Sedona, Arizona, the pristine greenery of New Zealand, the ancient landscapes of South Korea, and the unspoiled wilderness of rural British Columbia. Immersed in these environments, you can enter your inner quietude and interact with the earth's restorative power to release emotional and physical tension. Various on-site nature meditations, dynamic energy trainings, and heart-opening interactions will unfold new possibilities for you.

GETTING STARTED

Location

No specific location is necessary for Body & Brain Yoga training. It can be practiced indoors or outdoors, in your office, at a rest stop when you need a break during a long road trip, or even when you're sitting in a car or on a plane. To enjoy maximum benefits from Body & Brain Yoga, however, it's good to have a set place to practice. Choose a quiet location with little noise and enough space for stretching. Also make sure that the temperature is neither too hot nor too cold.

Clothing

Wear comfortable attire that doesn't inhibit movement. Clothes made of a natural fiber that are absorbent, lightweight, and breathable are recommended. It's a good idea to train without shoes, if possible. Nonslip yoga socks are helpful for holding postures and maintaining balance.

Time

It's best to train an hour or two after eating. Body & Brain Yoga includes movements that bend the body forward or backward and twist it from side to side, so you might feel discomfort if you train on a full stomach. Training in the morning is a great way to kick off an energy-filled day, and training in the evening helps you unwind before bedtime. Choose whatever works best for you.

Try to set a fixed time for training, if possible—ideally, one to one-and-a-half hours. But if this isn't practical, you should train for at least 20 minutes. It's best to train every day, but if that's not possible, then two or three times a week is sufficient. Although this book will serve as a basic guide, the best way to learn Body & Brain Yoga is to get the instruction and guidance of a professional instructor at a Body & Brain Yoga Tai Chi center.

Mindset

Before beginning a Body & Brain Yoga session, set your worries and plans aside and commit to spending time with yourself. Maintain your inner focus throughout the session. You can also set a goal that you keep in mind each time, such as reducing stress or pain, becoming more flexible, or making healthier choices.

APPENDIX

RESEARCH

Several studies have been published using Brain Education techniques. Various effects have been shown, including improvement in mood, sleep, stress response, and cholesterol.

[1]Stress Reduction, Positive Affect, More Dopamine

A study by the Clinical Cognitive Neuroscience Center of the Seoul National University College of Medicine in South Korea, in collaboration with the Korea Institute of Brain Science, compared 67 people who regularly practiced Brain Wave Vibration with 57 healthy people who did not. Brain Wave Vibration practitioners were found to be less stressed and displayed more positive emotions. Stress factors such as depression, anger, and the manifestation of psychological symptoms in the body were also significantly less. On the other hand, blood levels of dopamine, a neurotransmitter involved in pleasure, reward, and fine motor control, was higher in the Brain Wave Vibration practitioners. In subjects who had practiced Brain Wave Vibration for three years or more, blood dopamine levels were higher for those with more positive emotional states.

Jung, Y. H., D. H. Kang, J. H. Jang, H. Y. Park, M. S. Byun, S. J. Kwon, G. E. Jang, U. S. Lee, S. C. An, S. J. Kwon. "The effects of mind–body training on stress reduction, positive affect, and plasmacate-cholamines." *Neurosci.Lett*. 479, no. 2 (2010): 138-42. (2010), doi:10.1016/j. neulet.2010.05.048

[2]Alleviation of Depression and Insomnia

A team of researchers from the University of London and the Korea Institute of Brain Science compared the effects of Brain Wave Vibration to those of Iyengar Yoga and Mindfulness training. Over five weeks, 35 healthy adults participated in ten 75-minute classes in one of these three training methods. Participants were assessed before and after the five weeks of classes for mood, sleep, mindfulness, absorption, health, memory, and salivary cortisol. While all the methods improved stress and mindfulness, both Brain Wave Vibration and Iyengar training also improved overall mood and vitality. Where Brain Wave Vibration stood out was in decreasing the time it took participants to fall asleep (sleep latency) and in lower scores on a measurement of depression.

Bowden, Deborah, Claire Gaudry, Seung Chan An, and John Gruzelier. "A comparative randomised controlled trial of the effects of Brain Wave Vibration training, Iyengar Yoga, and Mindfulness on mood, well-being, and salivary cortisol." *Evidence-Based Complementary and Alternative Medicine* (2012), Article ID 234713: 13 pages. https://doi.org/10.1155/2012/234713.

[3]Lower Cholesterol and Inflammation

This randomized, non-blind pilot trial conducted by researchers at the University of Brain Education and the Korea Institute of Brain Science examined how Brain Education meditation (BEM) affects the conditions of patients with hypertension and/or type 2 diabetes compared with health education classes. Forty-eight patients with hypertension and/or type 2 diabetes took either BEM or health education classes at the Ulsan Junggu Public Health Center in South Korea over the same eight-week period. At the end of the eight weeks, levels of low-density lipoprotein cholesterol (LDL) had significantly decreased in the BEM group but not in the health education group. The expression of inflammatory genes was also significantly less after BEM training, as well as self-reported anger, fatigue, and loneliness. Self-reported confidence, happiness, relaxation, and focus increased for those taking BEM classes.

Lee, Seung-Ho, Sun-Mi Hwang, Do-Hyung Kang, Hyun-Jeong Yang. "Brain education-based meditation for patients with hypertension and/or type 2 diabetes: A pilot randomized controlled trial." *Medicine* 98 (2019): 19. http://dx.doi.org/10.1097/MD.0000000000015574

GLOSSARY

A

Abdominal Breathing *See* Dahnjon Breathing. *p. 131*

Ahmun \ ä-moon \ An acupressure point between the first and second vertebrae at the base of the neck. *p. 36*

B

Baekhwe \ bĕk-hwĕ \ An acupressure point at the top of the head. *p. 35*

Belly Button Healing A form of acupressure and abdominal massage centered on the energy point at the navel (Shingwol point). *p. 143*

Body & Brain Yoga A holistic health and mind-body training program that combines deep stretching and rotation exercises, meditative breathing techniques, acupressure methods, and energy awareness training. *p. 13*

Brain Education The five-step body-brain method of self-development on which Body & Brain Yoga is based. *p. 20*

Brain Education Healing Point (BHP) A tender or painful energy point on the body that facilitates healing when stimulated. *p. 141*

Brain Operating System (BOS) The key rules by which the brain runs, used for managing the brain. *p. 21*

C

Chakra \ ˈchä-krŭ, ˈshä-, ˈchŭ- \ A Sanskrit word meaning wheel or circle, referring to any of the body's seven internal energy centers. *p. 38*

Chest Breathing A breathing method designed to release tension through the loosening and relaxation of the chest. *p. 127*

Chi \ chē \ *See* ki. *p. 31*

Chun Bu Kyung \ chŭn-boo-kyŭng \ An ancient Korean scripture known as The Heavenly Code, explaining the trinity of Heaven, Earth, and Human. *p. 123*

Chunbushingong \ chŭn-ʻboo-shĭn-gōng \ A Body & Brain tai chi form that expresses the meaning of the *Chun Bu Kyung* through the body. *p. 123*

Chunjikiun \ chŭn-jē-kē-oon \ Cosmic energy, the highest level of energy. *p. 32*

Chunjimaeum \ chŭn-jē-mäœm \ Cosmic mind, enlightened consciousness. *p. 32*

Conception Vessel An energy pathway (meridian) down the front midline of the body, called Immaek in Korean. *p. 32*

D

Daechu \ dě-choo \ An acupressure point located right below the seventh cervical vertebrae. *p. 36*

Dahn \dän\ A Korean word that means energy, vitality, and origin of life. *p. 13*

Dahngong \ dän-gōng \ The most basic type of Body & Brain tai chi, which is strong yet gentle. *p. 115*

Dahnhak \ dän-häk \ The original name of Body & Brain Yoga, literally meaning "the study of life energy." *p. 13*

Dahnjon \ dän-jŭn \ A center in the body where energy (ki) is accumulated. The word most often refers to the lower dahnjon, located in the lower abdomen. *p. 38*

Dahnjon Breathing A breathing method designed to accumulate energy in the lower dahnjon, an energy center in the lower abdomen. *p. 131*

Dahnjon System The interrelated system of seven dahnjons (energy centers) in the body, including three internal dahnjons and four external dahnjons. *p. 38*

Dahnjoong \ dän-joong \ An acupressure point in the center of the slight indentation on the chest associated with the fourth chakra or middle dahnjon. *p. 36*

Dahnmu \ dän-moo \ A form of spontaneous dancing that follows the natural flow of energy. *p. 103*

DahnMuDo \ dän-moo-dō \ A non-combative Korean healing martial art based on energy principles that includes tai chi forms, kicks, punches, and blocks. *p. 116*

Dokmaek \ dōk-měk \ *See* Governing Vessel. *p. 32*

E

Earth Citizen A steward of the earth who puts their identity as a citizen of the earth before national, cultural, or religious identity. *p. 28*

Earth Citizen Movement A movement in which Body & Brain Yoga practitioners participate to raise awareness of the need to take on an Earth Citizen identity to have peace and prosperity on Earth. *p. 28*

External Dahnjons Energy centers in the palms of both hands (*see* Jangshim) and the soles of both feet (*see* Yongchun). *p. 38*

G

Governing Vessel A major energy pathway (meridian) that flows up the back of the body, called Dokmaek in Korean. *p. 32*

Geumchok \ gœm-chōk \ A method of practice that means "detach from stimulation" that involves maintaining focus in spite of internal and external stimuli. *p. 54*

H

Hwe-eum \ hwĕ-œm \ An acupressure point located at the perineum. *p. 36*

Hongik \ hōng-ēk \ A traditional Korean concept meaning "widely benefiting." This is a founding value and mission of Body & Brain Yoga. *p. 20*

I

Ilchi Kigong \ ĭl-jē kē-gōng \ A form of Body & Brain tai chi that expresses the philosophy and principles of the progression from creation to education to civilization, using smooth, flowing movements. *p. 122*

Immaek \ ĭm-mĕk \ *See* Conception Vessel. *p. 32*

Indang \ ĭn-däng \ An acupressure point between the eyebrows, also called "the third eye." It is associated with the sixth chakra, or upper dahnjon. *p. 35*

Injoong \ ĭn-joong \ An acupressure point in the center of the indentation between the nose and the lips. *p. 35*

Internal dahnjons The three main energy centers, located in the abdomen, chest, and head. *p. 38*

J

Jangshim \ jäng-shĭm \ An acupressure point located at the center of the palm on each hand. *p. 38*

Jigam \ jē-gäm \ A meditative exercise to introduce and experience the awareness of energy. Jigam means "stop emotion." *p. 52*

Jikigong \ jē-kē-gōng \ A form of Body & Brain tai chi used to gather energy from the earth and activate and balance each of the three energy centers. *p. 121*

Jinki \ jĭn-kē \ Unlimited energy received through pure cosmic awareness and accessed through deep, mindful concentration on the breath. *p. 32*

Joongwan \ joong-wän \ An acupressure point located halfway between the bottom of the sternum and the navel that is associated with the third chakra. *p. 36*

Joshik \ jō-shēk \ A method of practice that means "control breathing" used to calm the mind. *p. 53*

Junjung \ jŭn-jŭng \ An acupressure point located on the scalp, between the hairline and the crown of the head. *p. 35*

Jungchoong, Kijang, Shinmyung \ jŭng-choong, kē-jäng, shĭn-myŭng \ One of the three main energy principles of Body & Brain Yoga practice. In essence, it means "Physical energy is filled, the energy body becomes mature, and spirituality is awakened." *p. 48*

Jungki \ jŭng-kē \ Limited energy acquired from outside nourishment such as food and air. *p. 32*

K

Ki \ kē \ The vital energy that circulates throughout the universe, the essence of every creation in the cosmos. *p. 31*

Kigong \ kē-gōng \ An energy training method consisting of a series of body postures combined with concentration and breathing for the purpose of health, personal development, or martial arts training. Also called qigong, chigung, and chikyung. *p. 141*

Kihae \ kē-hĕ \ An acupressure point about two inches below the navel on the surface of the skin, literally meaning "sea of energy." It is associated with the second chakra or lower dahnjon. *p. 36*

L

LifeParticle A concept of the most fundamental unit of life, encompassing matter, energy, and consciousness. LifeParticles are often visualized as golden or aquamarine particles of light. *p. 51*

Lower Dahnjon A major internal energy center located two inches below the navel and two inches inside the abdomen, associated with physical energy. *p. 38*

M

Meridian Exercise A type of exercise designed to open the body's meridian system and balance energy. Also called "Doin" exercise. *p. 66*

Meridian A pathway through which energy moves in the body. *p. 32*

Middle Dahnjon A major internal energy center located in the middle of the chest, associated with mental and emotional energy. *p. 38*

MindScreen A three-dimensional field of consciousness on which all mental activity takes place. The MindScreen is a space and channel through which LifeParticles move. *p. 105*

Myunghyun \ myŭng-hyŭn \ A healing phenomenon that occurs as the body struggles to regain balance, literally meaning "alternating brightness and darkness." It may include uncomfortable symptoms such as dizziness, body aches, coughing, stuffy nose, etc. *p. 56*

Myungmun \ myŭng-moon \ An acupressure point on the back, opposite the navel between the second and third lumbar vertebrae. *p. 36*

Myungmun Breathing A breathing practice for developing the lower dahnjon, focusing on energy entering and exiting through the Myungmun point. *p. 139*

N

Noeho \ nwĕ-hō \ An energy point where the back of the head protrudes the most. It lies between the Okchim points. *p. 36*

O

Okchim \ ōk-chĭm \ Two separate energy points an inch to either side of the slightly protruding point at the back of the head. *p. 35*

R

Relaxed Concentration The state of focusing on something while maintaining a relaxed body and mind. *p. 97*

S

Shim Ki Hyul Jung \ shĭm kē hyŭl jŭng \ One of the three main energy principles of Body & Brain Yoga practice, literally meaning "where consciousness lies, energy flows, bringing blood and transforming the body." More simply stated, it means "where the mind goes, energy follows." *p. 50*

Shingwol \ shĭn-gwōl \ An energy point at the navel stimulated in Belly Button

Healing. Shingwol means "palace of God." *p. 36*

Sundo \ sŭn-dō \ An ancient Korean philosophy and mind-body practice that aimed to create a state of harmony within a person, between people, and between people and nature. *p. 19*

Suseung Hwagang \ soo-sœng hwä-gäng \ *See* Water Up, Fire Down. *p. 43*

T

Taeyang \ tĕ-yäng \ Two acupressure points on the sides of the head, one on each temple. *p. 36*

Tai Chi \ tī chē \ An internal Asian martial art based on kigong principles and characterized by flowing movements. *p. 114*

U

Unkibohyunggong \ oon-kē-bō-hyŭng-gōng \ A fundamental form in DahnMuDo consisting of seven sets of postures. *p. 117*

Upper Dahnjon A major internal energy center located just above and between the eyebrows in the center of the brain, associated with spiritual and intellectual energy and awakening. *p. 40*

V

Vision Meditation A meditation technique for realistically drawing out a desired goal or state of being using positive thoughts, emotions, and imagery. *p. 105*

W

Water Up, Fire Down One of the three main energy principles of Body & Brain Yoga, called Suseung Hwagang in Korean. It describes healthy energy flow. *p. 43*

Wonki \ wȯn-kē \ Limited energy inherited through genetic information from the parents. *p. 32*

Y

Yeondahn \ yȯn-dän \ A practice of holding a pose for an extended period. *p. 55*

Yongchun \ yōng-chŭn \ An acupressure point on the sole of each foot, approximately in the center and just below the ball of the foot. *p. 38*

ACKNOWLEDGMENTS

Body & Brain Yoga Education would like to extend special thanks to:

Models	Erin Carter
	Aaron Daniels
	Stephanie Jasieniecki
	Jacob Inally
	Leanna Diane Richardson
Photographs	Paul Markow
	Hyosang Ahn
	Jordan Diamond
	Dmitry Rukhlenko
Translation	Daniel T. Graham
Design	Kiryl Lysenka
Editing	Michela Mangiaracina
	Nicole Dean
	Phyllis Elving
	Jiyoung Oh
	Hyerin Moon
	David Driscoll
Illustrations	Junghyun Sohn
Consultants	Sayong Kim
	Jinhyung Lee

RECOMMENDED READING

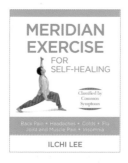

Meridian Exercise for Self-Healing

By Ilchi Lee

Alleviate common ailments as well as more serious conditions with this full-color, user-friendly book that identifies specific meridian exercises.

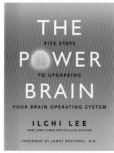

The Power Brain: Five Steps to Upgrading Your Brain Operating System

By Ilchi Lee

A user's manual for your brain that shows you how to use it to discover your value and improve your life through the five steps of Ilchi Lee's Brain Education method.

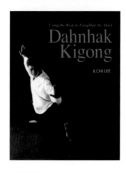

Dahnhak Kigong: Using the Body to Enlighten the Mind

By Ilchi Lee

This unique blend of mental and physical training was developed by Body & Brain founder Ilchi Lee. Kigong movements and focus will help you achieve strength and balance of body and mind.

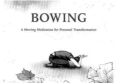

Bowing: A Moving Meditation for Personal Transformation

By Body & Brain Yoga Education

An ancient meditative practice is brought into modern times with step-by-step instructions and friendly illustrations. It can energize you and bring you closer to yourself.

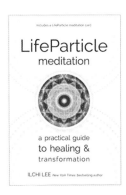

LifeParticle Meditation: A Practical Guide for Healing and Transformation

By Ilchi Lee

In this meditation book, targeted visualization techniques are provided for waking up the mind's abilities and making real changes in your health and your life.

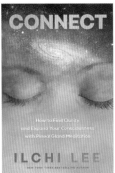

Connect: How to Find Clarity and Expand Your Consciousness with Pineal Gland Meditation

By Ilchi Lee

An inspirational guide to a powerful meditation method for opening the inner eye offers greater clarity about the health of your body, the dreams of your soul, and the wisdom of your spirit.

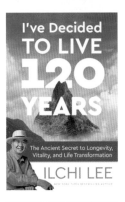

I've Decided to Live 120 Years: The Ancient Secret to Longevity, Vitality, and Life Transformation

By Ilchi Lee

The inspiration and practical advice found in this book can propel you to make the changes that will make it possible to live a long life full of vitality, passion, and purpose.

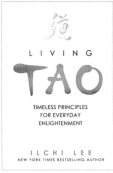

Living Tao: Timeless Principles for Everyday Enlightenment

By Ilchi Lee

This Tao teacher guides you to an understanding of the meaning of birth, death, and everything in between, building a foundation for living a complete life.

TRAINING TOOLS

Belly Button Healing Kit

This kit has everything you need to thoroughly experience the benefits of Belly Button Healing. It includes the Belly Button Healing wand, book, and online course. The wand is ergonomically designed to be comfortable to hold and to minimize stress on the neck and shoulders. Its three different-sized ends allow different amounts of pressure to be applied for different comfort levels.

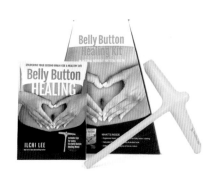

BHP Finder

The BHP Finder is specifically designed for BHP Energy Healing. Made of brass, this is a convenient tool to carry around to relieve tension and stress from the body and mind anytime, anywhere. The smaller end finds Brain Education Healing Points (BHPs) on the head, fingers, and toes, while the larger, rounded end presses and massages them.

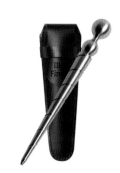

Hantoryum Qi Socks

Hantoryum Qi Socks are nonslip socks that help stabilize posture during yoga and other physical activities. These socks are lined with specks of Hantoryum, a mixture of rich, energizing earth metals that promotes proper energy flow, energy clearing, and grounding. Hantoryum inhibits most of the bacteria commonly found in closed footwear. The sock bottoms have anti-slip rubber dots.

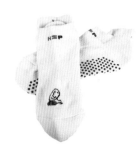

Bird of the Soul Essential Oil

A unique aromatherapy blend of 17 different oils developed by Ilchi Lee, Bird of the Soul Essential Oil opens the chakras, especially the fourth (heart) and sixth chakras (third eye). This can be used as a simple pick-me-up or as an enhancement for meditation.

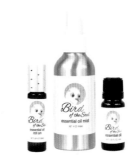

LifeParticle Card

The size of a business card, the LifeParticle Card is a meditation aid featuring the LifeParticle Sun image. This image of Sacred Geometry can be used for energy meditation and as a way to receive and send energy when you are on the go. Looking at the shapes and colors can bring the mind into a meditative state.

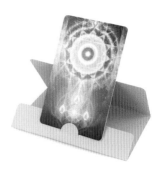

HSP Wooden Pillow

As used in Asia for hundreds of years, this round wooden pillow can be applied to any part of the body to relieve tension, pain, energy blockage, and fatigue. Made of sturdy, light paulownia wood, the HSP Wooden Pillow can also enhance abdominal circulation for improved digestion and overall well-being. It comes in small, medium, or large sizes to accommodate any height.

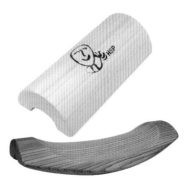

You can find these training tools at a local Body & Brain Yoga Tai Chi center, on ChangeYourEnergy.com, or on Amazon.com.

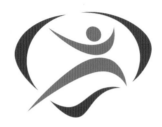

Find a Body & Brain Yoga Tai Chi
center near you at
BodynBrain.com
(877) 477-9642